WINNING
the food fight

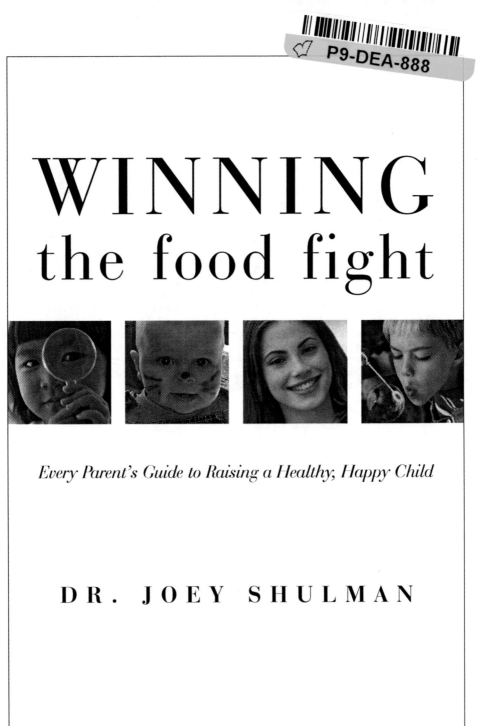

Every Parent's Guide to Raising a Healthy, Happy Child

DR. JOEY SHULMAN

⊛WILEY

John Wiley & Sons Canada Ltd
6045 Freemont Blvd.
Mississauga, Ontario
L5R 4J3

National Library of Canada Cataloguing in Publication

Shulman, Joey
    Winning the food fight : every parent's guide to raising a healthy, happy child / Joey Shulman.

Includes index.
ISBN 0-470-83249-5

    1. Children—Nutrition. I. Title.

RJ206.T63 2001   649'.3   C2003-900257-8

Production Credits
Cover and text design by Sharon Foster Design
Cover photograph/illustration by TK

Printed in the United States

10 9 8 7

WINNING
the food fight

This book is dedicated to my parents and family whose constant support allowed my light to shine. Without their continual love and encouragement, this project could not have become a reality.

Table of Contents

Acknowledgments

THERE ARE MANY people who have helped me on my journey. With their encouragement and help, this project was made possible.

Thank you to Robert Harris and John Wiley & Sons Canada, whose belief in *Winning the Food Fight* from the very beginning inspired me as a writer and gave me the motivation to continue. A very special thanks to my editor, Joan Whitman, for her expertise and unwavering patience in answering my countless questions. Your dedication was integral in bringing this information to the reader.

My deepest gratitude to Randy Taylor and cfrb 1010 Radio for giving me the opportunity to educate listeners on preventative health care. Randy, your passion for nutrition and genuine commitment to health care provided me with the forum to bring this message to the public.

To Stewart Brown, Lisa Chisholm, Sam Graci, and the rest of the ehn inc. family for their belief in me from the start and for their dedication in furthering preventative pediatric health care.

To my patients, listeners, readers, and fellow integrative health care practitioners, I express my gratitude. It takes courage to be open-minded about what was once deemed "alternative health care" and apply it as a preventative tool in your family's life. Bravo for your efforts to find a path to health and wellness.

As far as friends go, I am blessed to have the best. Thank you to all of my "girls" for picking me up and dusting me off whenever necessary.

To Mom, Dad, Danny, Sarah, Laina, Jamie, and "the boys," thank you is not enough, but they are the only words I have. Family has always been the special gift that has provided me with the necessary faith.

And, finally, thank you, Fred. Thank you so very much. I never dreamed it would be as good as it actually is.

I hope the words in this book reach parents and influence the health of our children.

This above all: To thine own self be true
—WILLIAM SHAKESPEARE

Introduction

As parents we must understand that children do
not belong to us. We are simply on a journey together
and have been entrusted with the responsibility
to guide them.—ANONYMOUS

THE TIME FOR change starts here! There is nothing more precious in life than our children. No effort is too large and no amount of money is too much when providing them with the best physical and mental health. Proper schooling, vacations, hockey games, ballet lessons, tutoring, and, of course, our love and attention are all essential in raising well-balanced children. There is another key component that is necessary to ensure a lifetime of health, vitality, and energy for them—it is the quality of the food they eat. A child's daily nutritional intake affects every aspect of their lives. Susceptibility to illness and infection, behavior, physical activity, performance in school, and mood are all affected by diet.

As your children grow, proper nutrition and exercise are essential for meeting the needs of their developing minds and bodies. Research clearly demonstrates that the food we give our children is by far the most powerful healing tool we can use on a daily basis. There is no medication, supplement, puffer, pill, lotion, or potion that can match the health benefits achieved by proper nutrition. In addition to helping the body fight off infection and disease, food can also be used as a very powerful preventative measure. Fresh vegetables and fruits, wholesome grains, and proper proteins are all essential in ensuring the health of your children's immune systems. Keeping their systems strong can prevent sickness from developing in the first place. Whether it is a toddler who is first starting to walk, or a teenager entering university, every meal is another opportunity to provide life-building nutrients ensuring a lifetime of optimal health. The time to get serious about making nutritional changes for you and your family is now!

My motivation for writing *Winning the Food Fight* was prompted by seeing numerous children suffering from poor health unnecessarily. Parents were unaware of the faulty nutritional choices that triggered or exacerbated their children's underlying conditions. I used to cringe every time a young patient entered my office with a stimulant drug to control behavior, such as Ritalin, in one hand and a sugary drink in the other. Why didn't the doctor tell him or her about the immune-suppressing and behavior-altering effects of white sugar? Shouldn't this information be made available to every parent? Shouldn't parents be made aware of the connection between food, mood, and physical health? As my private practice continued to grow, I started to focus more on the quality and quantity of food children were eating. By implementing nutritional therapies, I began to see and document phenomenal health improvements in the pediatric population. Recurrent bronchial infections, rashes, obesity, allergies, and asthma were all clearing up as irritating food selections were removed and replaced with healing, wholesome ones. In certain cases I would recommend vitamins or minerals that were lacking in a child's diet to accelerate the healing process. After seeing these dramatic health improvements, I realized how important it was to investigate the role of nutrition and its affect on a child's health. Today's obese child will become tomorrow's diabetic, heart attack, or stroke victim. A child with frequent ear infections and repetitive antibiotic use may develop irritable bowel disease or asthma. The child on Ritalin to treat attention deficit disorder may become addicted to drugs such as marijuana or cocaine in the future. It was time to inform parents of the natural options available to them.

Accessing healthy food for our children is harder than ever before. The food in our grocery stores is a far cry from the quality of food once eaten by our ancestors. In ancient times, the soil was rich with life-sustaining minerals, fruits and vegetables were clean and fresh, and grains were whole and rich in fiber and nutrients. Today, our soil is depleted of minerals, fresh fruits and vegetables are doused with herbicides and pesticides, and grains are refined and processed. To make things worse, a new technology has been developed to produce heartier, longer-lasting foods.

Terminology such as "genetically modified" and "biotechnology" are the latest catch phrases used to describe how the laboratory is now interfering with nature and our food chain. It is now possible to purchase a tomato that has been mixed with a fish gene. In truth, the splicing and dicing of DNA to form "newer" and "more beautiful" food has unknown health implications. I wish the problems stopped here, but they don't.

The increase in serving sizes has also created dangerous health problems. Children now consume larger amounts of food than ever before, and are dissociated from their internal hunger signals. "Bigger is better" and "two for one pizza" attract consumers, young and old, into fast-food establishments throughout North America. Because of the overindulgence of the wrong foods, adult diseases such as Type II diabetes, obesity, arteriosclerosis, and high blood pressure are now escalating to epidemic rates in our youth. We no longer have the luxury of waiting for double-blind research experiments to prove what we already know—nutrition can be your children's key to health!

In addition to the deteriorating quality of food and ever increasing serving sizes, parents must also deal with the clever ads promoting the latest unhealthy products their children are begging for. These ads are everywhere—on television, billboards, the back of cereal boxes, and even in schools! Do you know that pop machines are now in most school cafeterias? The easy access to this sugary soda means that children are likely to toss out their homemade, nutritious lunches in favor of their favorite pop.

Advertising companies are quite sharp and spend millions of dollars zeroing in on their greatest consumers—our kids! Chocolate bars at the checkout counter are even located at the eye level of every child! Coincidence or clever marketing?

The labeling of food has also become a confusing science for most parents to interpret. As consumers, we place our trust in commercial products. If a product claims to be "low fat," "filled with real fruit," or "a smart healthy choice," we expect it to be exactly that. Unfortunately, on closer inspection, many of these processed, packaged foods lack nutritional value and are major contributors to the diseases now plaguing our young. Unless they happen to have a degree in food chemistry, it has become difficult for parents to distinguish what is healthy and what is not. This book will help take the mystery out of label reading by clearly outlining what is health promoting versus what is health defeating for children's developing systems.

Although I have just outlined many of the difficulties involved in feeding children healthy foods, don't worry. Healthy eating can be achieved quite easily if the desire is there. Even in our fast-paced, processed world, parents can implement a nutritious, immune-enhancing diet for their children, whether they are tots or teens. Luckily, children often respond to even the smallest nutritional changes. A child is typically more in tune with his or her body, knowing that health, vitality, and healthy eating are part of their birthright. Keep a close watch on your children's behavior, energy, and moods as you start to implement a healthy diet. You will soon discover the positive healing effect that food can have. Of course, as the adult and the one in charge, the effort it takes to make a change in your family's diet falls on your shoulders. At first it will likely take a bit more effort, time, and concentration. However, with a little education, some motivation, and slight creativity, you will feel a great sense of peace and satisfaction knowing that you are providing your children with the best nourishment inside and out. Once you become accustomed to healthier food choices and options for your children, it will soon become part of your normal routine. As one of my obese pediatric patients said after shedding 15 pounds, "You were right, doc. Health is pretty cool!"

The diet-disease-illness connection deserves the attention of every parent, doctor, and child. It is the parents' right and duty to become active participants in ensuring their children's wellness by becoming knowledgeable about nutrition. Only then can we take the necessary steps to solve the problem. *Winning the Food Fight* clearly outlines easy nutritional tools that will facilitate a lifetime of health and wellness for the entire family. Whether the problem is as mild as an ear infection or as serious as Type II diabetes, this book provides you with the information on how to use nutritious food as the first line of defense against illnesses and as a road map toward wellness.

My goal in writing *Winning the Food Fight* is to provide you with easy-to-understand and applicable information on using nutrition as the primary tool to either "jump-start" or maintain optimal health in your children. You can learn all the information necessary to make the connection between the food your children eat and the state of their health. All children are different and not every suggestion in this book will work for every child. For each nutritional recommendation made, I have provided several tips that will help you find a "nutritional fit" for even the fussiest eater. *Winning the Food Fight* addresses the physical, biochemical, emotional, and "kid factor" issues of food.

Use this information in whatever way it serves you best. Within these pages you will find:

- An explanation of the optimal macronutrients your child requires on a daily basis (carbohydrates, fats, and proteins)

- Health consequences of sugar and other monsters such as refined flours, pesticides, aspartame, caffeine, and food coloring; natural, non-toxic alternatives will be provided

- The link between nutrition and obesity, Type II diabetes, attention deficit disorder, allergies, asthma, and gastrointestinal disorders (irritable bowel disease, Crohn's disease, and colitis), as well as foods that can assist in healing and reversing these illnesses

- Strategies to achieve "megahealth" in your children

- A list of healthier products available and how to shop in an affordable and nutritious way

At the end of each chapter, I will provide you with tips on implementing healthier eating patterns for your children in a section called "Try." These tips will range in order from easiest to hardest to implement. This system will allow you to take small steps when making nutritional changes while seeing the positive results in your children's health. Check out the Try section

I dedicate this book to every parent, grandparent, teacher, and caregiver who is committed to providing children with the best shot at a healthy future. I applaud all readers for picking up this book and moving in the direction of nutritional empowerment. You have officially taken the first of many steps toward improving the quality of your children's lives by improving the quality of their food. May we all eat well!

DR. JOEY SHULMAN

PART I

Getting to the Bottom of It!

When health is absent
Wisdom cannot reveal itself,
Art cannot be exerted,
Wealth is useless and Reason is powerless.
—HEROPHILIES, 300 B.C.

TO ADDRESS ANY problem, the contributing factors must be identified before solutions can be implemented to create balance and harmony. Of course, the health of our children is no exception to this rule. From a mild runny nose to severe asthma, the quality and quantity of the food children eat is the most powerful influence on their health. This section clearly identifies the nutritional contributors that have the potential to wreak health havoc on any child. Once the problems have been identified, foolproof methods of "winning the food fight" in your family will be provided. It is possible to ward off sickness and disease while getting your children excited about eating healthy, nutritious food. Read on!

CHAPTER 1

Food Fights

ARE YOU READY? Sure you are. From sweet tooth junkies, to fussy eaters, to the obese child, this chapter will help you discover that healthy eating and enjoyment of food can go hand in hand at any age. Easy, effective changes in and outside the home will be given as options to implement into your daily regime. I will show you how to shift from the old processed favorite foods to new, whole, live foods that promote health, proper growth and development, energy, and vitality. Let's get started.

WHAT IS YOUR FOOD RELATIONSHIP?

Does this scenario sound familiar to you? "Mom, can you please buy me a gumball?" Jimmy's mom always buys him a gumball. "Please, Mom, please!" Worn out and exhausted at the end of the day and desperately wanting to avoid a food fight with your child in the checkout aisle, you cave in. What does this typical, seemingly harmless scenario have to do with the state of our children's health today? Everything!

Ironically, while healthy eating is starting to receive more attention, the quality of food in our supermarkets has taken a plunge. Wholesome grains, fresh produce, and clean drinking water have largely been replaced with refined flours, packaged goodies, and sugary sodas. Studies clearly demonstrate that these foods can weaken a child's immune system, eventually reaping havoc on overall health. There is only so much nutritional abuse a child's body can handle before it collapses, surrenders, and starts to send out red flag signals. These red flag signals are what doctors refer to as symptoms. Symptoms are the language the body uses to speak to us. "Um, hello? Are you listening to me?" says the body. "If you continue to feed me harmful chemicals and nutritionally void food, I have no choice but to let you get a cold!" Symptoms may start off as subtle signs such as fatigue or a skin rash. However, if the underlying nutritional deficiency is not taken care of, these symptoms may develop into more serious conditions. It is disturbing but true that researchers are now finding fatty plaque developments in the arteries of children as young as age three! The connection between our continual consumption of nutritionally void food and the decline in the health of our young can no longer be swept under the carpet. As an old professor of mine said, in terms of food and health, "What can you expect? Garbage in, garbage out."

In conventional medicine, medicating children to eliminate symptoms of illness has become a common, accepted practice. Instead of investigating the root cause, antihistamines, antibiotics, and anti-inflammatory drugs are routinely prescribed to cover up any signs of underlying problems. Of course, there are definitely situations—such as bacterial infections or emergencies—when certain medications are warranted. However, often times the origin of the problem is overlooked. A medication's cessation or suppression of the body's natural response does not necessarily mean that health has been restored. Rather, it means the symptom has been eliminated. Unfortunately, when Western doctors "cure" a child of an ailment, nutrition is often the last area to be addressed. Doctors receive extensive pharmaceutical training, but a mere three hours of training on nutrition. As most parents have discovered, nutritional education is not often discussed during the average doctor's appointment. This reality means that caregivers must educate themselves about the connection between health and food.

In the past few decades, more and more research has demonstrated the role of nutrition in the maintenance of health and the prevention of disease. Although millions of people are starting to pay attention to the value of proper eating habits, the connection between childhood nutrition and health is largely overlooked. Foods can be used as a powerful healing tool or, if abused, an accelerator toward the breakdown of the body. There really is no better life insurance policy you can "buy" your children than a wholesome, nutritious diet. The first step in beginning your journey toward nutritional empowerment starts with your awareness. What is the state of your children's health? Do they suffer from frequent ear infections? Runny noses? Coughs? Are they overweight? How many times have they been on antibiotics in the past year? Do they suffer from behavioral disorders? Even if your children do not seem to have any health problems or symptoms of illness, proper nutrition is the best line of defense against future ill health.

YOUR RELATIONSHIP WITH FOOD

Prior to implementing changes in a child's health, I urge adults to take a look at their own relationship with food. What does a healthy lifestyle mean to you? Kids tend to imitate others. If mom or dad overeat, so will a child. Conversely, a young girl may mimic her calorie-conscious mother who constantly weighs herself and criticizes her own body image. In order to shift our kids back to a state of health and wellness, it is important to ensure that we are sending them proper messages about food and diet. Start by taking an honest look at your current state of health. Is there anything you can change? Providing yourself with healthy food choices and fresh water is one of the best ways to teach your children about honoring themselves. Raise the bar on health and wellness by taking an honest look at yourself and take action. Do you usually gobble down a low-fat muffin and a coffee every morning? Are you more inclined to grab processed, packaged food as a snack instead of a fruit, some vegetables, or whole grains? We can't expect our children to make the health changes that we ourselves have not made part of our own lives. If there are health changes you have not yet made or emotional links with food you have not dealt with, start now! You will be amazed at the difference that small steps toward health can make in your family's lives in a short amount of time. Once you begin to feel the improvement in energy, vitality, and mood, you will realize the results are worth the effort.

> *"Kids learn more from example than anything you say. I'm convinced that they learn very early not to hear anything you say, but watch what you do."*
> —JANE PAULEY, *journalist*

EXCUSES, EXCUSES, EXCUSES

"There is no more sincere love than the love of food."
—BERNARD SHAW

Dietary changes are difficult to make and can be even harder to maintain. If children learn proper eating principles at a younger age, the change will be much easier and longer lasting. People have strong attachments to food that extend far beyond taste. An individual's diet and eating patterns can be affected by numerous components, including emotions, cultural background, tradition, and societal influence. Before starting people off on the path of nutritional empowerment, I often ask them what obstacles have prevented them from making the necessary health changes. Without identifying the roadblock, nutritional changes are less likely to last. Does it have to do with a busy lifestyle? Religious restrictions? Lack of motivation or education? If the roadblocks can be identified and dealt with, there will be nothing to prevent your children from reaping the benefits of healthy eating. Over the years of speaking with parents about the importance of nutrition, I've heard countless reasons why they have not made any changes in their family's diet. The two most typical ones are: *"Thanks, but my child already eats a very healthy diet."* or *"Oh, those dietary suggestions couldn't possibly work in my family!"*

Let's take a closer look at some familiar excuses.

"Thanks, But My Child Already Eats a Very Healthy Diet"

In practice, I used to ask the question, "Do you feel your children eat healthy on a day to day basis?" I've stopped asking this because, without fail, the response was always a resounding "Yes!" The reality is that we all think our children eat relatively healthily. However, I have never met a parent or a child who could not benefit from making major dietary changes or from fine-tuning what they eat. Often parents are not aware of the chemicals and food irritants their children are consuming. Also, remember that everyone's definition of healthy eating differs. What might appear as a plateful of nutrition to one parent looks like a load of preservatives, food dyes, and sugar to another.

Most really believe that they are buying and preparing healthy, nutritious food for their children. Their hearts are in the right place, but, in today's world, unless you have a degree in nutrition, it is very difficult to distinguish health-promoting foods from "health–grabbers." What may appear and even smell like nutritious selections packed with vitamins and minerals can be loaded with anti-nutrients that can cause harmful effects in the body.

Anti-nutrients: Health Robbers on the Loose!

Unlike nutrients that provide a child's body with essential building blocks, *anti-nutrients* such as preservatives, food dyes, chemicals, and "funny fats" are health robbers that can wreak havoc on your children's systems. Boxed cereals, processed breads, crackers, muffins, ketchup, margarine, and luncheon meats are a few of these bandits. Chemicals such as MSG (monosodium glutamate), BHT (butylated hydroxytoluene), BHA (butylated hydroxyanisole), and sugar can all end up in your grocery cart and in your children's tummies without your awareness or consent. These chemicals leave little room for life-sustaining building blocks such as minerals, vitamins, essential fatty acids, and proteins, which are all necessary for optimal health. Even worse, these anti-nutrients have been linked to serious, life-threatening diseases such as cancer, Type II diabetes, asthma, and obesity. *Winning the Food Fight* will tell you about what should and shouldn't end up in your grocery cart.

Giving You the Whole Holistic Picture

The emphasis throughout this book will be on *holistic nutrition*—natural food sources that will provide positive nutritional health benefits in the body without creating negative side effects. It is important to remember that at its most fundamental level, food is intended to fuel the body and prevent premature breakdown. Cultural festivities, family gatherings, emotional enjoyment, and "breaking bread" with another are all wonderful reasons for eating, but are secondary to health and energy.

In addition to eating the wrong foods, children are also eating the same foods. Ask any youngster you know what his or her frequent favorites are and you're bound to get a list like this:

- pizza
- hot dogs
- hamburgers
- grilled cheese
- milk
- candy
- macaroni and cheese
- french fries

Sound familiar? Where are the fruits, vegetables, wholesome grains, nuts, and seeds? Isn't it a little disturbing that most of these foods are processed, refined, contain food coloring, or are drowned in sugar. As you will discover in Chapter 10 on allergies, the body does not tolerate eating the same foods over and over again. It needs a variety of several different types of fresh, live foods to live up to its potential. It is typically the "favorite foods" (the ones eaten five to seven days out of the week) that your children will eventually become sensitive or allergic to.

> *When fried vegetables are excluded, 30 percent of children consume less than one serving of vegetables per day.*

Food sensitivities and/or allergies are the underlying problems in many illnesses such as asthma, obesity, and behavioral disorders. Even children who are assumed to be eating a "very healthy diet" often benefit from a few changes.

"Oh, Those Dietary Suggestions Couldn't Possibly Work in my Family!"

This frequent excuse never fails to make me smile. I hear parents dismiss the idea of a healthy diet, assuming their children would never "go for it." Why does this make me smile? Those same parents show up in my office a few weeks later, proud to report that their children are enjoying the delicious new tastes of nutritious food. Children are flexible and will eventually respond to various changes, nutritional or otherwise, if a parent is loving, firm, and consistent in making these changes. The key to successfully implementing a healthy diet in your children's lives is to follow the rules of replacement behavior. For example, if you are eliminating a favorite food, such as a sugary delight or cheese, it must be replaced with another food item that is equally appealing or the change will not last. If you suspect a child is reacting to the food coloring in a Popsicle, why not replace it with a delicious homemade frozen treat made with natural juice? If a child develops ear infections from dairy products, but desperately wants some ice cream, try dairy-free soy or rice ice cream, which is equally delicious and now widely available. With today's advanced food technology, there are many delicious food replacements available.

This is the key: if children do not receive a replacement food that is equally enjoyable, they will start to feel deprived of the "old" food and will likely discontinue eating the new foods. Before convincing yourself that your children will not go for new foods try them! With consistent effort, tasty replacements, and a positive approach by parents, kids will quickly respond to new healthy foods that will create long-lasting health benefits. Even small dietary changes in a child's daily food regime, such as increasing water consumption and decreasing sugary juices, can produce beneficial health effects within a short time. The positive response in their energy level and sense of wellness will increase their enthusiasm for more healthy food changes. While it is true that some kids are especially finicky eaters, I have seen even the most stubborn kids respond positively when nutritious foods are presented in a creative, appealing way. Remember, you are the adult and therefore in charge of what your children eat. You are *not* doing them a favor by continually giving them processed, microwavable fast foods. These foods will only hinder the development of their health. Trust me—there is no better payoff than watching your children grow and develop into vital, energetic adults. Once health changes, such as weight loss, extra energy, or the disappearance of acne, become evident, children too will become excited and active participants in becoming nutritionally empowered.

The two excuses outlined earlier are the most common ones I encounter, but there are several more. Do any of these ring a bell?

"I Don't Have the Energy or Time to Change the Diet of My Whole Family"

After I make nutritional recommendations, patients often politely reply, "Thanks, but between the kids and work, I just don't have the energy or time to start." You too may feel that you can't muster up the energy to start, but, low energy or lack of vitality in you or your children is precisely why you can't afford *not* to start. Fatigue is often one of the first indications that a child's nutritional intake is insufficient. Learning healthy eating habits and stocking your cupboard with nutritious selections will initially take more time and concentration, but will soon become routine for the entire family.

"It Is Too Expensive!"

Eating healthily does not have to be an expensive venture. Although certain selections such as organic produce and antibiotic-free meats are more expensive choices, the family food budget can be balanced out by purchasing healthy grains, legumes, nuts, and seeds in bulk form. When comparison shopping, fruits and vegetables are always considerably cheaper than the average processed, packaged treat. In addition, cooking wholesome meals at home is not only healthier, but a much cheaper option when compared to eating out. I always point out to parents that days missed at work and medications are not cheap either! Please refer to Appendix II: Healthy Bulk Bargains for some money-saving ideas.

"My Children Cannot Stick to a Diet"

It is no secret that childhood obesity is occurring at epidemic proportions. Over 50 percent of children are now diagnosed as overweight and obese. As you will read in Chapter 8 on obesity, I am not in favor of putting children on a diet. For most children, a "diet" is likely to feel too restrictive and will therefore fail. This will lead to resistance and resentment toward any and all healthy changes. Instead of focusing on wellness, the idea of dieting can have a backlash effect, causing a child to gain even more weight, which will lead to even worse health and low self-esteem.

The statistics on diet and success rates clearly show that in both adults and children, over 90 percent of all diets fail. The diet industry is not a multibillion-dollar industry because it is working, rather because it is *not* working! It would be ludicrous to place children on a high-protein meal plan, a regime that involves drinking a shake for lunch or extreme calorie restriction. These methods will fail and will make your children miserable at the same time. Greater success will always be achieved by encouraging nutritious eating and by making a variety of delicious, nutrient-dense foods available to kids. Clinical studies show that weight loss is achieved not by eating less food, but by eating different food. By including some of the foods and food exercises recommended throughout this book, your children will be healthier and leaner. Weight loss success in children does not require more willpower, it requires more information.

"What If They Stop Eating?"

The parents of finicky eaters often resist making dietary changes for fear that their children will refuse to eat and lose far too much weight. While it is true that children might protest or be fussy when new foods are first introduced, this resistance will not last long. As the caregiver and the grocery shopper, you have the greatest influence on your children's well-being. If you have decided to stock your household with health-promoting foods, it is important for you to be loving but firm in standing by that decision. No whining, begging, or crying should make you budge. Remember, providing them with high-quality nutrition is one of the most loving things you can do. Try to introduce new foods into their diet with a calm and easygoing attitude. Kids will pick up on your stress or worry and will respond to it. As long as you are providing a variety of nutritious food options, you have nothing to worry about. Children are eager to learn as much information as possible. Educate them on the benefits of the food you are purchasing and invite them to become active participants in filling the grocery cart and table with wholesome food choices. With so many options to choose from, a child's resistance usually lasts no longer than a couple of days. With open communication and discussion, an agreeable and nutritious alternative is always found.

If your children do not like what you serve them, it is best to provide one or two healthy options. If they still do not want to eat, do not force them. They will soon ask for a healthy snack.

"My Child Has a Sweet Tooth That Just Won't Quit!"

Often parents report that their children suffer from a nonstop craving for sweets. Unfortunately, many parents are more inclined to indulge their children's cravings in order to avoid a full-blown temper tantrum. In addition, some feel it is better for their children to eat the wrong foods than to eat no food at all. *This notion is wrong and can create further complications in a child's health.* Of course, you can't let your children go hungry, yet indulging their cravings is a one-way ticket to health problems such as allergies, asthma, and obesity. In most children and adults, cravings are usually an indication of a biochemical imbalance that

"As a busy mother of three active boys, I realize that changing eating habits doesn't have to be the 'all or none' principle. Small changes, such as avoiding white flour and sugar, have had a significant impact on all three of my children's lives. Of course, this change is a learning curve and a continuing process. That said, I am pleased to report that my children have welcomed healthy eating as a part of our new daily regime."

—M. SIROIS, Oakville, Ontario

results from eating too many anti-nutrient and preservative-laden foods. As you will discover in the following chapters, there is a difference between merely enjoying the taste of food and actually craving it. Most people enjoy the sweetness of fruit or the taste of the occasional goody. However, cravings are an intense response to a withdrawal of a certain substance, such as sugar. This results in tantrums, irritability, headaches, "brain fog," and fatigue. It has been my experience that once a child is shifted back to a state of optimal health, cravings subside. Certain nutritional tricks of the trade, such as supplementing with vitamin C chewable tablets and drinking plenty of fresh, distilled water, can help a child get over the "sweet tooth syndrome." Check out Chapter 7 for more on this topic.

IT'S A FAMILY AFFAIR

As the gatekeeper of what your children eat, it is important to take a close, honest look at their diet and yours. The fact that you are reading this book is an indication that you are highly motivated to become nutritionally empowered. Before you make a change, let us examine the starting point of your family's nutritional status. Open your fridge to note exactly what is inside. Is it filled with healthy foods such as fresh produce, high-quality proteins, and wholesome grains, or are there frozen fish sticks, processed cheese, and microwave pizza? In order to start making a dietary change, it is crucial to know where the weaknesses are. The family fridge is one of the best indicators.

It doesn't matter if you are a family of five, a single mom or dad, or a grandparent. Start the shift toward health as a team—invite your kids to join in and participate in the fun. Whether it is exercising, eating less processed and fast food, or drinking more water, the entire family will benefit.

When introducing a healthier lifestyle for you and your family, it is wise to implement new changes at a gradual pace. This approach is more likely to have longer lasting results in children. However, if a child is suffering from an illness or disease, all harmful foods should be eliminated immediately. More serious issues such as childhood diabetes, asthma, obesity, and gastrointestinal diseases will be dealt with in later chapters.

When deciding which steps to take first, it is best to sit down as a family and create a family health goal list. Getting your children involved is half the battle. Explain to them the importance and effectiveness of goal setting. Whether the topic is health, finances, or career, writing down goals and actually accomplishing them teaches children an invaluable lesson. Goals that are written down and visualized have a much greater chance of achieving success and becoming a reality. As an added bonus, a family discussion about health goals will also open up the lines of communication, allowing your children to express how they feel about their bodies, their health, and the food they eat. Having their ideas considered will empower children, making them feel like active participants in the new and positive changes that are about to be made.

If your children are too young to be part of the discussion (i.e., under the age of three), start by writing out your own health goals. Your own positive nutritional changes will benefit the health and wellness of your children. Once completed, stick this list on the refrigerator and implement each goal one by one. When each goal is achieved, check it off the list so the entire family can share in the feeling of accomplishment and satisfaction.

When first creating your goals, try to make them as specific and measurable as possible. For example, include time frames or numbers. Some sample goals are:

- We will eat one more fruit or vegetable per day.

- The entire family will switch from drinking sugary juices to fresh, clean water for the next month.

- All members of this family will eat three meals a day. Skipping breakfast is not a good option!

- The children of family _____ will agree to take a healthy lunch to school at least three times a week instead of eating a pre-packaged, preservative-laden meal.

- We will eliminate white, refined bread and pasta from our cupboards and replace it with dense, grain breads and pastas that are high in fiber and have more protein.

- In order to shed excess pounds, all family members will stop munching on highly refined snacks such as chips in front of the TV. We will substitute with healthier snacks such as vegetables, fruits, nuts, or seeds.

- The entire family will go for a half-hour walk after dinner five times per week.

The goals that you and your family set are individual and specific to your family's needs. Luckily, our bodies are incredibly forgiving and will respond quickly to proper care and nourishment—"children's bodies respond especially quickly." Often implementing one small step toward health creates a dramatic increase in energy, strength, and vitality. Once this occurs, you and your children will be motivated to move on to the next health goal on your list.

Because I Love You

Food is intimately linked with emotion—there is no separating the two completely. Many parents, with the best intentions, use food to show their love and affection for their children. If a child is sad, has been teased at school, or is going through a hard time at home, parents often offer a piece of cake or cookie to make him or her feel better. If children do not act up at grandma's house, they are rewarded with candy. Of course, as you will read in the next section on the "80–20 rule," this situation is bound to happen occasionally and is impossible to avoid. However, when sweets or other food items are continually given to show affection or deprived for discipline purposes, a child's relationship with food and what it represents will change. For example, in a young child's mind, a cookie or a piece of cake may be equated with an emotion or an idea such as "Mommy loves me." To them, there is a double reward: *(1) the cookie taste good* and, *(2) the cookie feels good because of the emotion it represents.*

The problem arises when a child is sad and mom is not around to help, hug, or make everything "all better." Consciously or unconsciously, a child will begin to associate eating a sugary food with feeling better. These emotional associations with food, developed at a young age, can continue for a lifetime and are often the most difficult to conquer.

I strongly believe that using food for discipline will have negative consequences on children's health. According to Lean Birch, a psychologist at Penn State University, "There are things parents do with the best of intentions that turn out to be counterproductive. Using desserts to bribe kids into eating nutritious food can backfire. If kids are given one food as a reward, they will learn to prefer that food. They will also learn to feed the vegetables to the dog!" Healthy food is a right, not a privilege, and therefore should not be dependent on good behavior. Refer to Chapter 8 for alternative methods of discipline that do not involve food.

Until children reach a certain age, the responsibility of implementing a wholesome diet for them is the job of adults—the moms, dads, aunts, uncles, teachers, and caregivers. For the most part, adults are entrusted with deciding the quality of food that children will eat. Due to all the potential effects of food—both physically and emotionally—this is not a job that can be taken lightly. If the body, like a car, is expected to perform to the best of its ability, we must provide it with the highest quality fuel available. Eating wholesome foods at home teaches children invaluable lessons that will influence who and what they will become. It is important to explain to children that you are not a mean or overly strict parent just because you give them the highest quality nutrition and eliminate toxic foods from their diet. Instead, it is because you love them and want only the best for them. When we provide our children with the proper nutrition, we are sending them a message of love and respect. We can feel good about providing them with the nourishment that will feed their minds and bodies and pave a path toward future health. Compromising children's health by caving in and giving them a sugary delight is a big no-no that will cause more problems in the future.

THE 80–20 RULE

There is definitely a pleasurable and fun aspect to food and eating that cannot and should not be ignored. Food is one of the great joys in life, and I encourage adults and children to relish in the satisfaction and excitement a good meal or snack can offer. Eating for health and eating for pleasure do not have to be mutually exclusive. Fresh, wholesome sources such as whole grains, organic fruits and vegetables, and naturally sweetened goodies are just as delicious (or even more so!) as the preservative-laden treats found in most grocery stores today. Not only will wholesome foods tempt your children's palate, they will also result in optimal health. Unfortunately, marketing campaigns and food technology have steered children away from healthy eating and toward processed foods. Most children in North America today eat too much chemical food that has been covered up with sugar to mask a lack of taste. To add fuel to the fire, certain preservatives and taste enhancers (such as monosodium glutamate), which are in many food products, prompt children to eat more and more even if they are not hungry. Not only do our children eat the wrong foods for their young bodies, they also lose touch with their internal hunger cues and end up overeating. In order to reverse this effect and reawaken their taste buds, healthier food sources and fresh water must be introduced. Once your children's diet has been cleaned up, fruits, vegetables, and whole grains will actually begin to taste better. They will no longer be a chore to eat, but foods that your children will request.

> *The person who eats beer and franks*
> *With cheer and thanks*
> *Will probably be healthier*
> *Than the person who eats sprouts and bread*
> *With doubts and dread.*
>
> —JOHN ROBBINS, *Diet for a New America*

It is important to remember that it is impossible and unrealistic to expect your children to eat healthily *all* the time. As children grow older, adults lose a certain amount of control over the quality and quantity of the food they eat. Because this situation is inevitable, it is important to pick your battles instead of entering into a full-blown food war. For example, if a child is home for breakfast and dinner, make sure these two meals consist of healthy, flavorful selections. If lunch is eaten elsewhere, try packing a lunch for your children instead of allowing them to purchase processed foods and soda. The effects of practising healthy eating habits at home will overlap into other areas of their lives when you are not there to control the situation.

This is where the 80–20 rule is very effective. Try to have your children eat healthily 80 percent of the time and let them indulge in "kid stuff" 20 percent of the time. Unless a child is ill, this breakdown will still ensure health and wellness. If your children eat wholesome foods most of the time, but lapse occasionally at birthday parties, sleepovers, or vacations, that is perfectly okay and unavoidable. The nutrition that you give them at home will allow them to have the occasional "anti-nutrient" food without wreaking too much havoc on their young bodies. Healthier systems will have the strength and capacity to quickly recognize and eliminate sugary treats, chemicals, and the occasional fast foods that children indulge in. As important as proper nutrition is for our young, I also feel very strongly about preserving a child's self-esteem. There are times when it is better to allow your child to have a piece of birthday cake than to deprive him or her in front of other children. Kids do not like to feel isolated or different from their friends at any age—it is just not cool! When their friends are in your home, or when you are dining together as a family, proper nutrition should be expected. When the occasional ice cream cake shows up at a bowling party, let them eat it and enjoy it. You can undo the nutritional damage with fresh water and healthy food selections that evening or the following day.

Another helpful method for balancing out a "junk food day" is to add a nutritional fortifier into a child's daily regime. In my practice, I often refer to a product called greens+ kids (found in most health food stores), which contains an organic mixture of over twenty-five fruits and vegetables. This purple, berry-flavored powder is a very effective way to give children the nutritional value of whole, live foods. On poor diet days, double the servings of greens+ kids (i.e., an extra serving at dinner) for added protection.

It is important to take all areas of a child's life into consideration. Nutrition, emotional involvement, relationships, play, and socialization are all critical aspects that contribute to a child's healthy and well-balanced development.

At the end of each chapter you will find a section entitled "Try." This section outlines how parents can take the information in a chapter and put it into action. The steps outlined are ranked from easiest to hardest. Depending on your personality, you may be a "stick your toe in the water" or a "dive right in" person. It is up to you. I recommend starting with step 1 and moving down the list at a pace that is comfortable for you and your family. In the following chapters, the Try section will become more specific to certain food products, diseases, and illnesses when appropriate. Good luck!

TRY

1. Taking an honest look at your fridge and cupboards to see where you can start making nutritional adjustments.

2. Approaching food changes in a positive manner. Kids will pick up on your attitude and mimic it. Healthy food can be delicious and fun!

3. Making the necessary health changes in your life to provide a good example for your children to follow.

4. Making dietary changes a family affair. Ask your children for their "food feedback" to get a sense of their opinions, likes, and dislikes.

5. Removing food bribes from your discipline tactics. Start using other non-food options such as special time with mom, gold stars, or a movie night as rewards for good behavior.

CHAPTER 2

Far from the Land

As A CHILD, I naively believed that there was a large governing council or board that ensured public safety in all areas, including our food sources. There were laws restricting consumption of foods that could lead to the development of dangerous cancers, hardening of arteries, or obesity, weren't there? Cigarette packages have warnings on them such as "Smoking causes cancer" and "Smoking can harm your baby," so why do potentially harmful food products offer no such precautions? Where are the labels warning the public about the effect of hydrogenated fats on the health of your arteries? Why isn't monosodium glutamate (MSG) listed as a potentially toxic substance that can produce pituitary tumors in the brain? I've yet to find a refined floury product in the grocery store that proclaims its link to Type II diabetes. I feel it is my right to know if the genetic makeup of the fruits and vegetables I am feeding my family has been altered. I wish I could say I was exaggerating, but I am not. Labeling certain food products with health warnings may sound silly or overly dramatic when in fact, it may not be that absurd of an idea. Medical science is well aware that certain foods and chemicals are linked to the development of serious cancers, heart conditions, and other illnesses, yet the public is not being properly informed. Sadly, as I continued to delve deeper into the world of nutrition and food manufacturing, I quickly discovered that, for the most part, the responsibility of ascertaining food quality and safety lies in the hands of the consumer. It is up to us to research how much toxicity exists in the food we purchase at the local grocery store.

With food coloring, genetic modification (also called biotechnology), petroleum waxes, and pesticides becoming the norm in food production, assuring the safety of the foods you feed your child may seem impossible. However, with the proper guidelines it is not. There is a way to filter out most of the unwanted chemicals from your home. With more information, books, government involvement, and pressure from parents, food quality and safety can and will change. With continual pressure on the "powers that be," the use of toxic elements in our food, on our land and animals, and in our water sources will no longer be acceptable.

WHO IS TO BLAME?

It is evident that there are serious safety gaps in the way food is produced and monitored today. In addition, the emphasis that the medical community places on the value on nutrition and its link to health is minimal. In order to correct and reverse the problem, we must first identify the contributing factors that threaten the future health of our children. Presently, there are three major factors:

1. Food technology and manufacturing
2. Food additives and proper labeling
3. Lack of nutrional education in our medical system

Let's take a closer look at each of these factors:

1. Food Technology and Manufacturing

In the past fifty years, technological developments have been remarkable. Food technology is no exception. Our local grocery store stocks bigger and more colorful produce year round. Preservatives and refrigeration techniques now make it possible to extend the shelf life of some foods for over two years. Yet taste and appearance are not the only things to consider. We should also think of the costs to our health that result from potentially dangerous manipulations of food. It is our right to ensure that our children will not become the guinea pigs for future generations.

With every positive comes a negative. The positive is that North Americans now have a wide variety of food items to meet everyone's dietary restrictions and taste. Lactose-free, sodium-free, calcium-fortified, kosher, non-dairy cheese, and low-fat meats are all wonderful food options the public has to choose from. On the downside, certain current methods of food production have created foods that are drastically different from their true, natural forms. An apple grown in organic rich soil by a local farmer is far different from an apple grown with herbicides, pesticides, coated with wax to preserve its color, and then shipped halfway across the world. As a general rule, the further a food is from its original source, the less beneficial it is for us. Another example demonstrating the downside in food production is the method in which grains are now processed. The standard practice of milling and stripping grains to make refined flours for cereals, breads, and pastas, strip away precious vitamins, minerals, and fiber that are crucial for optimal health. To make things worse, these refined white flours enter a child's bloodstream far too quickly and can wreak havoc with blood sugar levels. Check out Chapter 4 and you'll see that carbohydrates and milled and refined flours are partially responsible for the increase in childhood obesity. Instead of eating fresh, live foods such as fruits, vegetables, and whole grains, children are more likely to snack on sugary cookies, white bread, or cheese-flavored crackers shaped like fish. Never before have we seen so many refined, processed food products on our grocery shelves labeled as fortified. Fortification of foods is merely the manufacturers' poor attempt to add back the delicate balance of nutrition that has been stripped away during the refining process. In truth, it is much more complicated than merely adding back a couple of B vitamins here and there such as niacin (vitamin B3) or folic acid. It is virtually impossible to strip a grain and then try to make it whole again by adding certain vitamins. Foods that were once deemed "nutritional powerhouses," such as whole grains, are now nutritionally void, creating detrimental health consequences.

Hydrogenating vegetable oils is another example of how the "new" technology is used to make food tastier and last longer. The process of hydrogenation involves heating up oil to a very high temperature, thereby converting it into a spreadable food such as margarine. Scientists now know that this method of food production can produce serious consequences for the health of the heart and arteries at any age. As you will discover in Chapter 6, hydrogenation can result in dangerous "funny fats" called trans-fatty acids, which have the potential to create ill health in our young. In his book *Eating for Optimum Health,* Dr. Andrew Weil states: "I am certain that TFA's [trans-fatty acids] will eventually be found to be detrimental to health in many other ways as a result of their effects on membrane and hormone function. I believe they promote the development of cancer and degenerative disease, increase inflammation, accelerate aging, and obstruct immunity and healing."[1]

Genetic modification, also known as biotechnology, is another example of a "new" popular technology used to alter our food sources today. This process involves changing a plant's traits by inserting a single gene or two or three genes into a crop to give it new, advantageous characteristics. Although this process is relatively new, it is being widely used on most crops in North America. For example, approximately half of the American soybean crop planted in 1999 carries a gene that makes it resistant to an herbicide used to control weeds. About a quarter of US corn planted in 1999 contains a gene that produces a protein toxic to certain caterpillars, eliminating the need for certain conventional pesticides. Sounds like a perfect solution to promote food quality, doesn't it? In truth, the answer to this question is unknown. Long-term studies on the health hazards associated with genetic modification are unavailable, leaving scientists uncertain of potential consequences. Consider these comments by the following well-known researchers and doctors regarding the process of genetic modification:

- "The genetic modification of food is intrinsically dangerous. It involves making irreversible changes in a random manner to a complex level of life about which little is known. It is inevitable that this hit-and-miss approach will lead to disasters. It must disrupt the natural intelligence of the plant or animal to which it is applied, and lead to health-damaging side-effects." (Dr. Geoffrey Clements, leader of the Natural Law Party, United Kingdom)

- "The perception that everything is totally straightforward and safe is utterly naive. I don't think we fully understand the dimensions of what we're getting into." (Professor Philip James, author and director of the Rowett Research Institute, Aberdeen)

- "If it is left to me, I would certainly not eat it. We are putting new things into food, which have not been eaten before. The effects on the immune system are not easily predictable and I challenge anyone who will say that the effects are predictable." (Professor Arpad Passaic, Rowett Research Institute)[2]

When respected and famous broadcaster and geneticist Dr. David Suzuki was questioned about the safety of genetically modified foods, he simply said, "Any scientist that says it is safe is either very stupid or deliberately lying. The tests simply haven't been done."

A slightly disconcerting situation when it comes to the health of your child, isn't it?

The genetic modification of food is definitely picking up momentum and is being used without discretion. Consider the following facts:

- Genetically modified soybeans require two to five times more herbicides than natural soybeans.[3]

- The Canadian government does not require labeling of genetically modified foods.[4]

- There are about forty varieties of genetically engineered crops approved for marketing in the United States. As a result, 60–70 percent of the foods on your grocery shelves contain genetically engineered (GE) components.[5]

- Transgenic foods may mislead consumers with counterfeit freshness. A luscious-looking, bright red, genetically engineered tomato could be several weeks old and of little nutritional worth.

It is abundantly clear that the genetic modification of food is grossly under-researched with unknown health implications. Presently, scientists are creating absurd crossbreeds of genes, for example, that are resulting in crops that are completely resistant to herbicides due to genetic modification. Unfortunately, genetically modified (GMO) foods are not always properly labeled. The public needs to pressure the government to take proper action. The quality and safety of the food we are feeding our children should take top priority. Genetically modified "frankenfood" is not something that should end up in the systems of our young without our permission. I recommend taking action by getting in touch with your local health official and by purchasing products that are labeled non-GMO. Remember, the consumer is king. The greater the public demand, the more likely it will be that you will see non-GMO foods as common items on the shelves at your local grocery store.

2. Food Additives and Proper Labeling

The average North American consumes approximately 11 pounds of food additives per year as preservatives, colors, bleaches, flavors, emulsifiers, and stabilizers. To make matters worse, usage of pesticides and herbicides are at an all-time high and are now detected in our children's systems. Each of these chemicals is toxic, and scientists are unsure about how their interactions with each other may affect health. With the rising number in pediatric cancers, it is time to investigate the potential threat to our food by demanding that the amount of chemicals used in food production be minimized and made public. According to Kate Kempton, vice-president of Sierra Club of Canada: "Chemicals do not have the constitutional right to be presumed innocent until proven guilty. That's where the innocent children and others have the right to be protected from debilitating problems. The answer cannot be to spray blind and hope like hell the science we now have turns out to be wrong."

Consider some of the alarming statistics about the increasing amount of chemicals in our children's system:

- The food color tartrazine (yellow), found in drinks, cakes, snacks, ice cream, and confectionery, can cause asthma attacks and hyperactivity in children.

- Many ice creams contain a chemical called diethyl glucol, which is used in antifreeze and paint removers.

- The flavor enhancer MSG, found in drinks, candy, chewing gum, and soups, has been shown to cause migraines, blurred vision, behavioral problems in children, and difficulty focusing.

- Aspartame poisoning is cumulative—it builds up in your system and can affect nervous system functioning.

- Aspartame accounts for over 75 percent of the adverse reactions to food additives reported to the US Food and Drug Administration (FDA). Many of these reactions are very serious and can cause seizures or death.

- In the United States, the use of pesticides has increased thirty-three times since 1945.

- As a result of normal agricultural use, forty-six pesticides—some of them known to cause cancer or other harmful health problems—have been discovered in the groundwater in twenty-six states.

- A Swedish study found that an ordinary bag of potato chips may contain up to 500 times more of a chemical called acrylamide (a carcinogen) than the amount allowed by the World Health Organization in drinking water.

There are hundreds of other potential health threats caused by food additives and pesticides. These toxins pose even more of a risk in children because of their smaller stature and developing systems. This information is not being presented as a scare tactic. I want to arm readers with enough information to make proper health care choices. While it is virtually impossible to completely eliminate all chemicals from your children's food, it is quite possible to minimize their exposure considerably. To reduce the amount of chemicals in your home, start by becoming a label reader. As a general rule, if the words listed are difficult to pronounce or are more than eight letters long, that should be your first clue that the product does not promote health. The label "certified organic" ensures that the food is free from herbicides or pesticides and other drugs. Although these items are more expensive, the assurance that your children are not ingesting harmful pesticides, hormones, and antibiotics is well worth the cost. Products labeled "certified organic" means the food has been grown and processed for a minimum of three years without the use of harmful chemicals. Farmers who grow certified organic produce are regulated by strict standards, must keep thorough records, and have their farms inspected annually.

Unfortunately, aside from certified organic, labeling laws can be fairly loose and creative, often sneaking a chemical or food item into a product without the consumer's awareness. For example, suppose you are aware that your child is sensitive to MSG foods. It seems fairly logical to merely eliminate all products that list MSG on the label, right? Wrong. Many names listed on ingredient labels may be derivatives or even contain MSG. Words such as autolyzed yeast or hydrolyzed protein may contain the additive MSG. Unless a parent has a degree in food chemistry, how could he or she possibly be aware of this information? This common finding only further supports the argument that it is better to purchase most of your food from fresh, live sources and minimize the amount of packaged processed food you allow into your home.

When shifting your family back to the basics of nutrition, try to eat as close to the original source as possible. For example, crackers that contain refined flour, the preservative *butylated hydroxytoluene* (BHT), salt, and have a shelf life of two years are far removed from the original whole grain they once were. Try healthier alternatives such as raw nuts, seeds, legumes, and fresh fruits and vegetables. Whenever possible, try to shop locally to ensure your produce is fresh and alive. Have you ever noticed how you feel when you eat foods such as raw salads, fresh fruit, or whole grains? You actually feel more vibrant, energetic, and closer to optimal health. Because they are closer to their source, these foods offer benefits that are far beyond what the microscope or laboratory can measure or identify. As Dr. Dean Ornish, author of *Reversing Heart Disease*, says when referring to processed goods: "Unfortunately, a longer shelf-life for the product, may mean a shorter life for you!"[6]

3. Lack of Nutritional Education in Our Medical Schools

Education regarding nutrition and its link to health has received minimal attention in North American medical schools today. As mentioned in Chapter 1, the average medical doctor receives a mere three hours of nutrition training in total. In comparison, by the time you finish reading this book, your nutrition education, hour for hour, will be close to or more than that of the average medical doctor. Why do doctors overlook the undeniable connection between nutrition and health? There are several answers to this question. For starters, the standard medical approach is based on symptoms. If a patient has a cough, the symptom is treated with a cough suppressant. If someone has inflammation of the colon, an anti-inflammatory steroid such as prednisone is prescribed. If an artery is clogged, a surgical procedure can be done to remove the plaque buildup in the artery. If and when the symptom subsides through drugs or surgery, it is thought, for the most part, that health is restored.

> *"The role of the doctor is to amuse the patient while nature does the healing."*
> —VOLTAIRE

According to the allopathic model of medicine, the average patient has little or no responsibility for his or her own health, and the doctor searches for a "quick fix" when illness occurs. The focus is primarily on detection and treatment rather than prevention and maintenance of health. Of course, medications do have an important role in medicine. However, as a nation we are letting our health deteriorate and becoming dangerously dependent on drugs and doctors to restore our own wellness. Instead of a health care system, the allopathic model has shifted to that of a sick care system. Consider the description that Dr. Hitchcox, author of *Long Life Now*, gives of the typical heart attack patient:

> *Each year, nearly 400,000 Americans undergo heart bypass surgery from blocked coronary arteries. Most patients believe surgery will correct their problem. However, it is an immutable law of biology that a disease caused by a detrimental diet cannot be corrected by surgery. We ignore this principle at our peril. Following heart bypass surgery, 50% of arteries clog up within 5 years. Following balloon angioplasty, 33% of dilated arteries clog up within 4–6 months. Each heart bypass operation replaces only 6 inches of an arterial system leaving the other 60,000 miles of total length. In most cases, these procedures do not improve survival. By treating symptoms with drugs or surgery while ignoring the underlying cause, treatment often becomes an expensive exercise in futility.[7]*

As a society, we have become too complacent in accepting chronic diseases such as arthritis, heart disease, diabetes, and stroke, which are intimately linked with a poor diet. Instead of focusing on expensive detection techniques such as scans, X rays, and blood analysis to identify and treat a disease once it has already occurred, the focus should shift to education and preventative nutrition to ward off future ailments.

Peer acceptance is another reason why most medical doctors tend to shy away from nutrition and alternative medicine. Curiously, there is a perception that if a treatment is natural, it is deemed unscientific. It is not uncommon for a medical doctor with a holistic approach to be thought of as a "quack" or a "radical." Not wanting to be singled out, doctors are more likely to stick with traditional medicine than to practise differently than their colleagues. Fortunately, this notion is starting to change, albeit slowly. Now that many scientific journals and magazines such as *TIME* are publishing articles on nutrition and its link to health, the subject is getting more serious attention.

I applaud doctors who are taking the best from the medical model and combining it with a holistic and preventative approach. Not only will education and prevention save millions of health care dollars, it also enables patients to take responsibility by becoming more active in maintaining their own health. The model of health that combines science and nature to serve the patient best, is referred to as the *integrative model*. The integrative model of health (once called the alternative or holistic model) differs in its approach to health care. Integrative practitioners view the body as one intercommunicating system. The systems can be likened to that of an orchestra. When one instrument or system is not well tuned or absent, the entire piece of music or the entire body will suffer. Unlike a fast-acting drug that can eliminate a symptom immediately, the integrative model often occurs at a slower pace by focusing on healing the underlying problem. The goal is to prevent symptoms or disease from developing in the first place. On the whole, more time is spent with patients investigating all causes that can influence health—food, exercise, emotional stress, and lifestyle management. Under this scope of care, the enormous influence of nutrition on health is duly investigated. Medical doctors with an integrative approach may use standard diagnostic tools such as blood analysis or X rays in conjunction with nutritional and lifestyle therapies. If the health care practitioner is not a medical doctor (i.e., a chiropractor, naturopath, or nutritionist), depending on the area of expertise, other tests or therapies such as food allergy testing, hair analysis, chiropractic adjustments, or homeopathic remedies may be used. While taking the entire body into consideration, the goal is to shift an individual back to a state of optimal health using natural means to support—not suppress—the body's processes. Clean living and clean eating is a motto used by many practitioners who use the integrative model.

> *According to a recent study, nearly eight in ten Canadians take prescription drugs or over-the-counter pain medications such as painkillers, tranquilizers, and antidepressants in any given month. This widespread usage among Canadians aged twelve and older contributed to a total drug bill exceeding $15.5 billion last year (2001), up 8.6 percent from the previous year, and averaging more than $500 per person.*

Remember, when seeking the advice of any health care practitioner, medical or non-medical, it is your right to ask as many questions as you like regarding the practitioner's background, credentials, and the therapies recommended for you or your child. It is important for patients to do their homework on health and potential health care practitioners.

THE EARTH, OUR HOME

In addition to human health concerns, there are also environmental concerns that must be considered. We have become negligent with our environment and are creating dangerous, irreversible changes by the way we are producing food and chemicals. Deforestation, destruction of the ozone layer, and the greenhouse effect are all issues directly related to food technology. One of the greatest concerns that scientists and farmers face today is the poor state of our topsoil due to overharvesting of crops without proper care. In North America, the topsoil has been stripped down to such a degree that it is severely nutrient deficient, contributing to malnourishment and the development of disease. According to Bernard Jensen, author of *Empty Harvest*,

> *"Be gentle with the earth."*
> —THE DALAI LAMA

"Few realize that the current state of widespread soil erosion in North America threatens our way of life. It may seem hard to believe, but only a few inches of topsoil stand between you, me and starvation."[8] Scary, isn't it? Did you know that it takes 100 to 1,000 years to regenerate one inch of topsoil? I too was shocked when this fact was pointed out to me. These problems can seem insurmountable. So what can we do as individuals to take action and make positive changes in the environment? It all comes down to a bumper sticker I saw several years ago that simply stated, "Think globally, act locally." Showing children how to care for the earth as their "outside home" teaches them invaluable lessons about gratitude and respect. Recently, my five-year-old nephew taught me a very powerful lesson on remembering to care for the environment. Feeling lazy and tired at the end of the day (no excuse, of course!) and unable to find a recycling bin to discard my empty plastic bottle, I thoughtlessly chucked it into a trash can. Without skipping a beat, my nephew looked up at me and said with a straight face, "Auntie Joey, plastic is not for throwing out. It is to be used again and again. Don't you know that?" Of course I know that and, of course, instantly humbled, my hands were in the trash, picking out the bottle I had just discarded. At the wee age of five, my nephew was able to catch me in a lazy, thoughtless moment and remind me that it was important to do my part to take care of the earth.

There are several other ways we can teach our children to care for the earth. If children are taught to treat the environment with respect, it will automatically be second nature to them (no pun intended, of course!). Our children are the generation of the future. As important as it is for them to care and properly nurture their bodies with food and exercise, it is equally important that they learn proper care and appreciation for the environment. By teaching them about composting, recycling, and proper waste disposal techniques, they will learn to take pride in their world. As demonstrated by my nephew, these invaluable lessons will help to ensure a future world of healthy food, healthy land, and healthy air for their children in years to come.

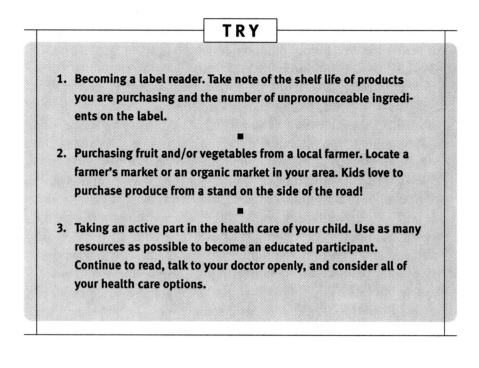

TRY

1. Becoming a label reader. Take note of the shelf life of products you are purchasing and the number of unpronounceable ingredients on the label.

2. Purchasing fruit and/or vegetables from a local farmer. Locate a farmer's market or an organic market in your area. Kids love to purchase produce from a stand on the side of the road!

3. Taking an active part in the health care of your child. Use as many resources as possible to become an educated participant. Continue to read, talk to your doctor openly, and consider all of your health care options.

■

4. Having your children learn about recycling at a young age. Allow them to separate and recycle the plastic from the paper products. Do not tolerate littering.

■

5. Taking an active role in protecting your children's food sources and the quality of their food in the future. Contact your local government official about what you can do to make a difference. Remember, you never know how far-reaching an effect your action will have.

NOTES

1 Weil, A. *Eating Well for Optimum Health.* (New York: Alfred A. Knopf, 2000.)

2 www.organicconsumers.org

3 www.organicconsumer.org

4 www.fishtomato.com

5 www.safe-food.org/

6 Ornish, D., Dr. *Dr. Dean Ornish's Program for Reversing Heart Disease.* Ivy Books, 1996.

7 Hitchcox, L. *Long Life Now: Strategies for Staying Alive.* Celestial Arts, 1996.

8 Jenson, B. & Anderson, M. *Empty Harvest.* Avery Publishing Group, 1990.

CHAPTER 3

Health from the Inside Out

H AVE YOU EVER wondered why your finger heals when it is cut? Platelets rush to the area to form a fibrin plug, which forms a scab, and the wound is shielded until new skin is formed. Scientists and doctors are able to explain the process involved in healing the cut with big fancy words, but they cannot tell you exactly *what* has healed your child's skinned knee. This mysterious healing capability is referred to as *innate intelligence*. With its innate intelligence, the body is constantly trying to maintain a healthy balance called homeostasis. For example, if your children are suffering from a bacterial infection, part of the homeostatic feedback mechanism creates a fever to kill off the potentially harmful bacteria. If they have eaten spoiled foods, the innate intelligence of their bodies will attempt to maintain a homeostatic balance by eliminating the foods through diarrhea or vomiting. Without the body's natural ability to keep things in check, harmful invaders like bacteria, viruses, toxins, and even food would wreak havoc on a child's health. Luckily, most children are born with innate intelligence mechanisms that keep their internal systems running smoothly.

Today children are exposed to a significant amount of toxins including pesticides, herbicides, food chemicals, sugar, caffeine, and salt. These numerous assaults on health can threaten their ability to maintain homeostasis, thus creating a significant amount of free radical damage. This occurs when cells are damaged through exposure to the toxins in the air we breathe, the food we eat, and the water we drink. It is virtually impossible to prevent free radical damage from occurring. However, it is possible to help counteract and minimize the damage in order to prevent sickness and disease. The top five ways to prevent or counteract free radical damage in our bodies are the following:

1. Consume plenty of antioxidant foods such as fresh fruits and vegetables.

2. Eliminate "funny fats" from your diet such as trans-fatty acids, fried foods, and margarine. (Please refer to Chapter 6 on fats for further details.)

3. Don't smoke.

4. Exercise a minimum of three to five times per week for a minimum of 1 hour.

5. Supplement with a high-quality multivitamin daily. Give your children their multivitamin with food for optimal absorption.

Even though we like to think of our bodies as invincible, there is only so much abuse the body can take before it starts sending out red flag signals. At first, these signals are subtle and often overlooked. We may not pay much attention to seemingly harmless signs such as a runny nose, heartburn, stomach aches, and bloating, or we might attribute them to the wrong cause.

Often parents claim that their children have a chronic runny nose because they are in day care with other children. While your child may have caught a bug while in day care, it would be wise to take a step back and examine the state of your child's immune system. Why is it that one child in day care will suffer from a cold while another will not? Of course, there are many answers to this question such as genetics, environment, and quality of food. However, prior to assuming these symptoms are normal, it is best to investigate all triggers that may weaken immunity.

THE BODY: MORE THAN THE SUM OF ITS PARTS

In most medical schools, doctors learn about the body by breaking it down into various components such as the immune system, the nervous system, the cardiovascular system, the digestive system, etc. Typically, each system is taught individually and in great detail. Although this method is fairly effective and thorough in terms of teaching, viewing the body as separate systems often influences how doctors practice. When one system is ailing, a doctor will treat that particular system without much thought to the other parts of the body. Simply look at our current medical model for evidence of this. If you are seeking medical assistance for your child, first you are sent to the jack of all trades health care professional called the general practitioner. If he or she is unable to assist, your child will then be referred to a specialist. Skin problem? Off you go to a dermatologist. Heart? The cardiologist is the logical choice. Frequent and unrelenting ear infections? A visit to an ear, nose, and throat doctor is likely. Instead of viewing the body as greater than the sum of its parts, the design of the current health care system treats our bodies as individual systems that do not overlap. This type of approach can send parents on a wild goose chase, going from doctor to doctor in an attempt to find out the root cause of their child's health problem.

Most medical doctors I work with are wonderful practitioners who treat their patients to the best of their ability. Unfortunately, the reality is that today's doctor is overworked and understaffed, making consultations with individual patients often too short to adequately address their needs. Communication from doctor to doctor about the various therapies and/or drugs prescribed for an individual patient becomes difficult. It is not uncommon for a busy doctor to give out a prescription over the phone without even seeing the patient!

The point is that when one system begins to suffer from ill health and the root cause is left untreated, other systems will begin to suffer as well. Instead of medicating or treating various symptoms, it is wise to step back and ask certain questions. What are the conditions that have led to the development of poor health? Are your children allergic to dairy? Are they stressed? Are they reacting to a food chemical you are unaware of? If the symptom is merely masked and the underlying problem is not addressed, the body will send out another symptom of distress from either the same or a related system.

Let's look at how a child's individual systems intercommunicate. Suppose a child is undergoing a stressful situation at home or in school, such as parental divorce, a failed test, or conflict in the schoolyard; such a child's nervous system would be under considerable strain. Chronic nervous system stress (often referred to as the fight or flight response) will create problems in other areas of the body. For example, it would not be uncommon for this child's immune system to also be affected by this stress, making the child more susceptible to harmful microbes that can cause an infection. To comfort the child, the mother might offer a white sugary treat such as a cookie or a Popsicle. As you will discover in the following chapters, certain foods such as white sugar suppress immune system function. The combination of emotional stress and anti-nutrient food such as white sugary treats will lower this child's immune system and increase susceptibility to an ear infection or bronchial infection. Now here is the kicker. The child is then put on antibiotics to clear the infection. Although antibiotics will rid the infection (only if it is bacterial), it will also destroy part of the vital "good bacteria" called microflora, which live in the digestive system and are critical to overall health. An unhealthy digestive system means poor digestion and the potential for future infections, thus creating a vicious cycle in this child's body. See the connection? One system influences the next. To ignore the interdependence among all the systems in the body would be foolish. Consider the following examples:

- Children who are not breast-fed (and whose immune systems and digestive systems may therefore be compromised) are more likely to suffer from asthma and allergies.

- An overweight or obese child is at risk of Type II diabetes.

- Twenty-five percent of individuals suffering from inflammatory bowel diseases suffer from arthritis.

THE KEY TO HEALTH: THE DIGESTIVE SYSTEM

As just outlined, all systems are critical to health. However, many doctors consider the nervous system to be the master of all systems. It controls breathing, the beating of our heart, walking, and proper brain function. Without its delicate control and smooth functioning, life would cease. However, in addition to the nervous system, there is a "copilot" master system—the digestive system—that can either tip the scales in favour or against health. It is impossible to achieve optimal health without optimal functioning of the digestive system. The digestive system performs three critical functions that maintain overall health in the body: (1) digestion, (2) absorption of nutrients, and (3) excretion of waste. When these functions do not run smoothly, a myriad of health problems such as the following can appear:

- Allergies
- Asthma
- Attention deficit disorder
- Colic
- Constipation
- Diarrhea
- Ear infections
- Eczema
- Enuresis (bed-wetting)
- Irritable bowel syndrome
- Obesity

Curiously, even people suffering from gastrointestinal disorders are often unaware of how their digestive system really works.

Typically, the status of a child's digestive system is examined only if there are obvious gastrointestinal problems such as constipation, diarrhea, bloating, and belching. Medical doctors rarely link the state of children's health with the way food is digested, absorbed, and excreted. For optimal health in your child, remember that HEALTHY DIGESTION = HEALTHY BODY. Often parents are perplexed by the link between intestinal health and symptoms in other seemingly unrelated areas of the body. I often see puzzled looks on their faces when they ask, "I don't understand. How can my child's asthma be linked to the intestinal tract?" It is a valid question. (For more information on allergies and asthma, see Chapter 10.) If a child is not properly digesting food because of poor enzyme secretion in the stomach, eating the wrong foods, or eating too much food, the body can perceive the food source as an invader and cause an allergic reaction. For example, undigested protein particles in milk can cause inflammation in the bronchial lining of a child's lung, resulting in an asthma attack. Once a child achieves proper digestive health, symptoms and adverse reactions subside. Consider the following facts that highlight the important link between proper digestive capacity and health:

- If food is not chewed properly, undigested food particles in the intestinal system can be perceived as invaders and attacked. This "attack" within the body can result in a histamine response (allergies), asthma, fatigue, and irritability.

- If a child is not breast-fed, the digestive system is not "sealed off" properly with the bacteria needed, which can leave a child more susceptible to the development of ear infections, bronchial infections, and allergies.

- Eczema, a common skin disturbance that appears as dry, itchy, and red skin, is often linked to food allergies. This response is often related to poor intestinal health.

- The dense amount of protein in cow's milk can be perceived as invaders by a child's immature intestinal system. These proteins can result in colic, ear infections, bronchial spasms, chronic rhinitis (runny nose), and irritability.

It is important to remember that all children are biochemically different. One child's digestive capacity will be different than another's. Child A may have a weak constitution, developing an infection from eating white, sugary delights, while child B shows no adverse reactions to the treat. Adults and children have varied genetic wiring. Those with a strong constitution and thrifty genes can eat whatever they like, never get sick, and never gain an ounce. I call such a child the "George Burns exception" to the rule. George Burns, a famous comedian and entertainer, lived to the ripe old age of 100, yet smoked a cigar daily, drank alcohol frequently, and ate an abundant amount of red meat. Aside from having a loving wife and family, it is likely that George also benefited from a stronger constitution and genetic makeup, which allowed his body to take more abuse than most. To determine your children's individual constitutions, ask yourself the following:

- Do they suffer from frequent colds, coughs, or ear infections?

- Do they experience wild fluctuations in mood or energy level (hyper/ extreme fatigue)?

- Do they take frequent medication (antibiotics, puffers, acne medication)?

- Do they have enough energy to participate in outdoor play, sports, and exercise?

- Are they overweight?

If you have answered yes to any of the above questions, chances are your children's diet could use a little fine-tuning.

Throughout this book I often refer to the health of the digestive system. Only by restoring the proper balance and integrity of digestion through the food we eat, the supplements we take, and the water we drink can optimal health be achieved. Even if your children are healthy, happy, and symptom-free, paying attention to their intestinal health when they are young can pave the path for a healthy future.

The Story of Digestion: The Health of Your Pipes

In order to ensure intestinal health in your children, it is important to have a brief description of how this system runs. Let's start Digestion 101.

The digestive system is a self-enclosed tube that begins in the mouth and stops at the anus. Surprisingly, the digestive process first begins in the nose! When the nose detects an appealing smell such as baked bread or a homemade meal, the brain is signaled to release saliva in the mouth. This step sparks the digestive system to start working and gets the body ready to break down the food it is about to receive. Throughout the digestive system, different sections secrete different enzymes. Enzymes are the catalysts that assist with the proper breakdown of food, which begins in the mouth with the secretion of the enzyme called salivary amylase. Salivary amylase breaks down starchy foods into smaller, more absorbable sugar units. Having your children thoroughly chew their food before it goes down the pipes is an essential step in the digestive process. Unfortunately, with today's fast pace at mealtime, many miss out on the first stage of digestion and gulp down large amounts of food that have not been properly chewed. This habit can be easily changed with a little extra focus when eating as a family at the kitchen table. Insufficient chewing causes children to overconsume food by disassociating them from their hunger cues (which signal satiation) and increases the risk of having large, undigested food particles end up in the stomach. Undigested food particles can be perceived as invaders (otherwise know as antigens) and can trigger a negative reaction in the body. How a child reacts to undigested food particles depends on his or her "weakest link" (i.e., lungs, skin, stomach). Encouraging your children to chew their food thoroughly is the first of many steps to improve and strengthen their digestive capacity.

After leaving the mouth, food travels through a long tube called the esophagus to enter the stomach. The stomach secretes two critical components that continue the digestive process: the enzyme pepsin and hydrochloric acid (HCl). Pepsin is responsible for the breakdown of proteins such as those found in meat, chicken, dairy, eggs, and soy. Proteins are broken down into smaller, more absorbable units called amino acid chains. Overloading the stomach with too much food or too many of the wrong foods can overtax this essential organ, impeding the entire digestive process. While the environment in the mouth is alkaline, the environment in the stomach is acidic because of the secretion of hydrochloric acid, which further assists with the breakdown of food and the absorption of minerals. Improper HCl secretion can result in malabsorption of vital vitamins and minerals that the body needs to function properly. Low HCl, otherwise known as hypochlorydia, can also cause heartburn, chest pains, gastric hernias, and stomach aches in a child or young adult. Because of the highly acidic environment, the stomach is lined with a mucous membrane for protection. Once food makes its way into the stomach, the stomach churns and churns, turning particles of food into a liquid called chyme. This key step is necessary for the food's next stop in the small intestine.

The small intestine is a 20–22-foot long tube and is lined with millions of villi, which move back and forth to absorb the broken-down nutrients into your bloodstream. In the small intestine, the digestive juices once again switch to an alkaline state where protein, fats, and carbohydrates are further broken down. The length of the small intestine is divided into three parts: the duodenum, the jejunum, and the ileum. According to *Dr. Jenson's Guide to Better Bowel Care*, "The small intestine is the site of approximately 90% of the absorption of nutrients into the bloodstream."[1] If this site of the digestive system becomes impaired by poor food choices, overconsumption of harmful chemicals, or overconsumption of food, proper absorption will not occur and a child is at risk of becoming nutrient deficient.

At the terminal part of the small intestine there is a valve called the ileo-cecal valve, which is normally closed, separating the food being absorbed in the small intestine from the bacteria in the large intestine. If this valve is not functioning properly, potentially harmful microbes that normally live in the large intestine can flow backwards into the small intestine and interfere with healthy absorption. The small and large intestine are completely different environments that perform separate functions. If the digestive system is working as it should, the two never meet. Keeping the ileo-cecal valve functioning properly by eating a high-fiber diet and drinking plenty of fresh, clean water is critical in maintaining overall digestive health.

The final stop on the food's journey down the intestinal tract ends in the large intestine and the rectum. The large intestine is 5 feet long and divided into sections called the cecum, ascending colon, descending colon, sigmoid colon, and rectum. Its main function is to complete the final digestive processes necessary for healthy elimination. The large intestine has the "good bacteria" called microflora, which is crucial for proper digestion and elimination. The large intestine is also responsible for the compaction of stool, which is eliminated by the anus.

FIGURE 3.1: The Digestive System

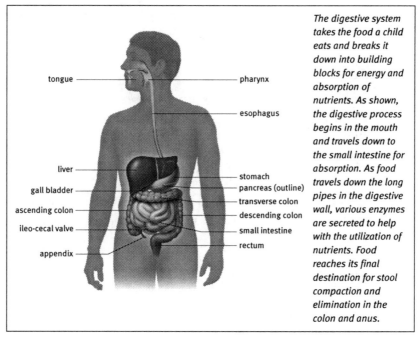

tongue

pharynx

esophagus

liver

stomach

gall bladder

pancreas (outline)

transverse colon

ascending colon

descending colon

ileo-cecal valve

small intestine

appendix

rectum

The digestive system takes the food a child eats and breaks it down into building blocks for energy and absorption of nutrients. As shown, the digestive process begins in the mouth and travels down to the small intestine for absorption. As food travels down the long pipes in the digestive wall, various enzymes are secreted to help with the utilization of nutrients. Food reaches its final destination for stool compaction and elimination in the colon and anus.

What Is Normal Excretion?

Equally important as proper digestion and absorption of nutrients is proper excretion. On average, a healthy colon will remove waste matter within eighteen to twenty-four hours. Infants and children have more frequent bowel movements—about one to four per day. A child should eliminate without strain, and the stool should be formed and have a brownish hue. Red or black stool is often indicative of various health problems and should be brought to your doctor's attention.

Parents often do not pay much attention to the regularity of their children's bowel movements. I frequently hear parents reporting that their children's bowel movements are normal and regular, and that they excrete approximately every two to three days. This is definitely *not* normal and must be addressed properly. Often a sluggish bowel is one of many symptoms that indicate poor digestive health, an overloaded system, and/or food sensitivities. If a child does not have a daily bowel movement, his or her system runs the risk of autointoxicating—that is, the body will produce toxic substances that may threaten health.

Some of the most common symptoms that accompany a poorly functioning excretory system are:

- Allergic shiners
  (dark circles under the eyes)
- Allergies
- Behavioral problems
- Constipation
- Dry skin or hair
- Ear infections
- Runny nose
- Skin rash such as eczema

If your children are not having regular bowel movements, some underlying causes may be food allergies, candida (yeast infections), recurrent antibiotic usage, and a diet that consists of refined flour and sugar products. The following chapters will address these causes in great detail.

SUPERBUGS

2000 BC: Here, eat this root.
AD 1000: That root is heathen. Say this prayer.
1850: That prayer is pure superstition. Here, drink this potion.
1940: That potion is snake oil. Here, swallow this pill.
1985: That pill is ineffective. Here, take this antibiotic.
2000: That antibiotic doesn't work anymore. Here, eat this root.

The two most common reasons for visiting the pediatrician are ear infections and respiratory infections. After a diagnosis, medical doctors commonly prescribe antibiotics to "squash the bugs!" Unfortunately, the overuse of antibiotics has created a dangerous scenario, leaving doctors with fewer options to choose from.

Most ear or respiratory infections are viral, not bacterial, in origin. Antibiotics have no effect on a viral infection. Unfortunately, even if a test is done to determine the bacterial or viral nature of a child's illness, the common practice is to put a child on antibiotics even before the lab results return. The indiscriminate use of these drugs is creating antibiotic resistance or, in other words, "superbugs" that are difficult to kill.

Surveillance figures by the Centers for Disease Control and Prevention show that resistance among S. pneumoniae, the bacterium that causes half of all ear infections, is approaching 50 percent in the United States.[2]

As with any medication, antibiotics are appropriate in certain cases. In acute and potentially life-threatening bacterial infections such as bacterial meningitis (inflammation of the meninges that line the brain), antibiotics have been quite a blessing. However, we are depending on these drugs for every ill, creating a problem we may not be able to control. It is prudent to look for other options. Preventative health care is one of the most effective steps to take, as it eliminates the need for antibiotics in the first place.

In addition to the superbugs that are developing resistance, there is another serious problem regarding the overuse of antibiotics. In the digestive system, antibiotics kill the good bacteria as well as the bad bacteria. Following a bout of antibiotics, children are left deficient in good bacteria, leaving them more susceptible to future illness. An overgrowth of candida (yeast) is a common occurrence with antibiotic usage. Candida overgrowth in a child or adult can result in headaches, fatigue, constipation, irritability, and allergies. Sounds like backwards medicine doesn't it? If your child has been on a recent dosage of antibiotics, following their use, it is essential to supplement with more of the good bacteria called acidophilus. (See Chapter 9 for more details on yeast.)

TRY

1. **Eating fruit alone.** By itself, fruit is incredibly cleansing to the body (especially when eaten in the morning, such as a fruit-filled breakfast). Eating fruit at the end of a meal (such as a dessert) ferments the other food that has just been eaten, making digestion sluggish.

   ■

2. **Having your children eat their last big meal by 6–7 PM.** Metabolism slows down as the day progresses. If your children ask for a late night snack, pick something nice and easy to digest, such as a banana, which will also help them sleep.

   ■

3. **Encouraging your children to chew their food well.** Remember, proper digestion begins with the act of chewing.

   ■

4. **Slowing down.** Do not overload the body with too much food in a short amount of time. Mealtime should last at least twenty minutes.

   ■

5. **Paying attention to the frequency of your children's bowel movements.** A healthy system should excrete without strain at least once a day.

NOTES

1 B. Jenson, *Dr. Jensen's Guide to Better Bowel Care* (New York: Avery Publishing Group, 1999).

2 www.detnews.com

PART II

Your Child's Nutritional Needs

Let food be thy medicine, and medicine by thy food.
—HIPPOCRATES

THE FOLLOWING THREE chapters review the categories of macronutrients—carbohydrates, proteins, and fats—necessary for proper growth and development in every child. For an easy-to-use menu plan that includes healthy meal and snack options, please refer to Appendix III. Take a look at the nutritional requirements and number of calories and note that they vary from child to child, with the averages estimated at:

- 1,000 calories per day for a one-year-old
- 1,300–1,500 calories per day for ages four to nine
- 2,000 calories per day by age ten

If your child is very active, please remember that as physical activity increases, so does the required caloric intake. Let's dive in and learn about what we should and shouldn't be putting on our family's plates.

CHAPTER 4

Carbohydrates and Kids

W HILE RESEARCHING this book, I surveyed a number of people on the topic of carbohydrates. The following are the questions that were asked and the most typical responses received.

Q: *What is a carbohydrate?*
A: *"Carbs" are breads and pastas, such as bagels, muffins, breads, and cereals.*

Q: *Is it essential to eliminate carbohydrates for weight loss?*
A: *To lose weight, it's best to keep carbohydrate intake to a minimum. Completely eliminating breads and pastas for a specific amount of time would help the weight come off more quickly.*

Although these answers were partially correct in identifying breads and pastas as carbohydrates, they were also missing some important information. There is a lot of confusion about carbohydrates and their necessity in the diet. Everywhere you turn, there is a new program or commercial advertising the perfect diet to "lose weight and feel great!" While most of these books, videos, and speakers have the best intentions in educating people on the principles of healthy eating, the public is still puzzled and frustrated about what constitutes the optimal diet. High protein, low protein, bread is okay, bread is not okay—people are throwing up their hands in bewilderment. Perhaps part of the problem is what I refer to as *nutritional information overload*—too many terms, too much chemistry, and not enough time in the day to read through several nutritional texts. I hope this book does the work for you by condensing nutritional information and focusing on the important stuff that busy parents need to know about their children's nutrition.

The other part of the problem is that in the field of nutrition, there are many opinions on what constitutes the perfect diet. One nutritionist or doctor may recommend food combining at meals (a method of combining different foods to enhance digestion), while another may think that eliminating breads and pastas is the best road to health. For example, recently certain carbohydrates have received some undeserving bad press due to the promotion of high-protein diets for weight loss. These diets promote eating high-protein food sources such as meat, chicken, fish, and dairy and drastically minimizing or eliminating grainy products such as breads, pastas, rice, cookies, and cakes. It can become quite confusing when trying to make sense of it all. The reality is, carbohydrates are not the food enemy—they are nature's greatest sources of fuel for the human body. In fact, carbohydrates are so integral to a child's growing system that approximately 50 percent of a child's total dietary intake should be derived from carbohydrates. It is healthy and necessary for children to eat complex carbohydrates including fruits, vegetables, high fiber breads, pastas and cereals. In addition to providing them with the cleanest-burning fuel available, in their wholesome form, carbohydrates offer essential nutrients such as vitamin B, fiber, calcium, and iron. As you will discover, the "carbohydrate problem" does not lie in the carbohydrate itself but in the refining and processing of the grains we consume.

GLUCOSE = GAS

Our bodies need fuel to run properly. Similar to the gas we put in our car, glucose is the fuel that keeps our system running smoothly. (A good way to remember this is the g for gas and glucose!) The body breaks down all carbohydrates into glucose, which is then transferred into the cells for energy. Certain parts of the body, such as the brain or red blood cells, can use only carbohydrates as an energy source. Other parts of the body can use other sources of fuel such as fat or protein, but none burn as efficiently and cleanly as carbohydrates. Young, growing bodies in particular require a constant flow of high-quality fuel to maintain energy and vitality. Children's high energy demands mean that they must eat several servings of nutritiously packed carbohydrates throughout the day. Contrary to many fad diets, proteins and fats are not suitable substitutions for carbohydrates on a long-term basis. Fats cannot be broken down into a proper source of fuel and proteins do not burn cleanly in the body, leaving behind a potentially dangerous residue called ammonia. Even if your children are overweight or obese, eliminating their carbohydrate intake is not the solution. Without the glucose from carbohydrates, the biochemical reactions in the body would eventually come to a halt, leading to organ failure and eventually death.

So, what exactly is a carbohydrate? Carbohydrates are derived from plants and can be found in fruits, vegetables, legumes, and grains (cereals, breads, pastas, rice, etc.). All carbohydrates are made up of sugars linked together. The number of sugars in a molecule determines whether the carbohydrate is classified as *simple* or *complex*. Simple carbohydrates have one, two, or at most three sugars linked together to form a molecule. They occur naturally in fruits, vegetables, and milk products, or in processed foods such as candy, honey, table sugar, syrups, and carbonated beverages. Simple carbohydrates with one sugar unit are called monosaccharides (mono = one). Examples of monosaccharides are:

- Glucose
- Fructose (fruit sugar)
- Galactose (milk sugar)

Disaccharides (di = two) are also simple carbohydrates that link together two sugars. Examples are:

- Maltose (glucose + glucose)
- Sucrose (table sugar) (glucose + fructose)
- Lactose (glucose + galactose)

Complex carbohydrates are the second category. These molecules consist of hundreds or thousands of sugar units linked together to form larger sugar molecules. Examples of complex carbohydrates are breads, cereals, starchy vegetables, legumes, rice, and pastas. Depending on the amount of processing and refining of the grain, complex carbohydrates can have either a high-fiber content (such as twelve-grain breads, spelt bread), or a low-fiber content (called refined carbohydrates, such as white bread, bagels, and enriched cereals). It was once thought that low-fiber, refined carbohydrates were empty calorie foods that neither helped nor harmed your health. As will be explained in the following section, research has now proven that this notion is false. These foods have become one of the great health robbers of our time, and are partially responsible for the dramatic rise in childhood obesity, Type II diabetes, and mood disorders.

There are four calories for every gram of carbohydrate consumed. As mentioned, it is recommended that active children derive approximately 50 percent of their total caloric intake from carbohydrates. For example, a child consuming 1,800 calories per day would require 225 grams of

Examples of Serving Sizes of Various Healthy Complex Carbohydrates

Food	Carbohydrate (grams)	Calories
FRUIT		
Apple (medium)	21	81
Banana	27	105
Orange	16	65
Orange juice	26	112
Raisins (½ cup)	79	302
VEGETABLES		
Carrot (medium)	8	31
Corn (½ cup)	21	89
Peas, green	12	63
Potato (large, baked, plain)	50	220
Sweet potato	28	118
Broccoli (½ cup), raw	2	12
GRAINS		
brown rice (½ cup)	50	232
Whole wheat bread (1 slice)	11	55
Cereal (1 cup)	24	110
Pasta (1 cup)	34	159
Cream of wheat (¾ cup)	20	96
BEANS		
Chickpeas (1 cup)	45	269
Navy beans	48	259
Pinto beans	44	235
Blackeye peas	22	134

carbohydrates (1,800 x 0.50 divided by 4 calories for every gram of carbohydrate) Of this amount, it is best to select most of your carbohydrate choices from the complex, high-fiber category.

THE PROCESSED PROBLEM: WHITE FLOUR

If you are a well-versed label reader, you have probably noticed certain words now listed on packaged products such as enriched, refined, bleached, processed, and fortified. Welcome to the world of refined foods, a method of food production that has become prevalent in our society and is falsely marketed as "healthy eating."

The expression "processed foods" is an umbrella term that refers to various manipulations of food including the addition of chemicals, herbicides, pesticides, waxes, coloring, genetic modification, and much more. In this section I will focus on one of the major problems affecting our children's health—the refinement of grains. While certain areas of food technology have made extraordinary advances, the advent of refined, milled flours is not one of them. Once you become aware of the prevalence of these refined goods, you will soon discover that most of the products in your local grocery store are filled with these nutritionally void, potentially harmful flours.

So, what exactly is the refining process? The refining process takes a whole food such as a grain and breaks it down into individual components. There are three parts to an individual grain: the endosperm, the germ, and bran. The endosperm contains mostly starch and protein; the germ is rich in unsaturated fats, proteins, carbohydrates, and vitamins B and E; and the bran contains a large percentage of fiber and moderate amounts of B vitamins. The refining process of a grain strips away the bran and the germ, leaving only the endosperm. This breakdown removes most of the nutritional value of the grain and upsets the important balance that previously existed between the three components. Since the processing of the grain eliminates much

> *Only 2 percent of the flour consumed in this country is whole grain. On average, twenty-four ingredients are removed during refining.*
>
> **Source: Healthy Kids: Help Them Eat Smart and Stay Active for Life by Marilu Henner. Regan Books, New York 2001**

of the natural sources of nutrition, manufacturers add back vitamins such as folate, iron, and vitamin A to cereals, breads, and pastas. This process is called fortification. Do not be fooled—replacing these vitamins synthetically through fortification does not make the grain whole again. It is impossible for the delicate and specific balance once created by nature to be perfectly restored. This was not the way we were intended to eat our carbohydrates.

The practice of refining grains started to gain momentum over the past few decades. Modern wheat has been changed drastically and is virtually unrecognizable from its distant, ancient grain relative. Today's wheat is not grown for its nutritional content, but to increase harvest and yield. In addition, the gluten content, a wheat protein, is much higher than it was in distant times, making it the perfect choice for the production of high-volume commercial baked goods. Researchers have speculated that the increase in the number of cases of celiac disease (a digestive disease where gluten cannot be tolerated, causing damage to the small intestine and interference with normal absorption of nutrients) may be linked to the high gluten content found in grainy products today. It is estimated that approximately 90 percent of current grains consumed—such as bagels, breads, pastas, cookies, and muffins—have been though a refining process. To the manufacturers of these products, the refinement of flour is very appealing because it can reduce cost and lengthen shelf life. Unfortunately, this type of manufacturing sacrifices the true flavor and nutrition of the grain in exchange for the mighty dollar. In his book, *Eating for Optimum Health*, Dr. Andrew Weil explains the advantage that modern millers felt was achieved from producing white flour:

> *Millers could produce this new food (white flour) much more cheaply than stone-ground flour, and it had a much longer life in storage. White flour made lighter, fluffier breads and pastries, and, being a product of new technology, seemed attractively modern. In Europe, city dwellers with sophisticated palates quickly came to prefer these new foods, while the old-fashioned, coarse, dark breads of the past were stigmatized as the fare of peasants and ignorant country folk.*[1]

Kids are the front-runners when it comes to eating refined products like sugary cereals, cakes, muffins, and cookies. Who can blame them?

Over the years, their taste buds have become accustomed to the "melt in your mouth," unnaturally sweet taste, and textures of these foods. For most children, nutritionally stripped down, milled flour is the only type of bread they have ever known. Have you ever noticed how many children love to take an entire piece of white bread, roll it into a ball, and pop it into their mouths whole? Stripped of all essential fiber and nutrients, white, mushy bread is a far cry from the original wholesome food it once was. As far as the body is concerned, eating white flour is the same as eating white sugar. Like sugar, refined flours (in the form of glucose) enter the bloodstream far too quickly. This surge of glucose creates dramatic fluctuations in blood sugar levels, leading to a number of potential symptoms in kids such as mood fluctuations, weight gain, increased risk of future heart disease, lack of energy, and constant cravings. We must examine the potential health costs these flours may pose on the future health of our children. According to Dr. Bateson-Koch, author of *Allergies—Disease in Disguise*:

> *When consuming an excessive amount of refined foods, nutrients stored in the body must be utilized to metabolize the sugar packed into these processed foods. When these nutrients are depleted, an alternate pathway in the body must be used, creating an imbalance in the body's biochemistry. This imbalance results in altered signals to the brain leading to cravings and addictions.*[2]

Children's cravings often manifest as irritability, moodiness, sadness, whining, hyperactivity, and complaints. This sort of behavior leads to an anxious, unpleasant environment for both parent and child. Nevertheless, giving children another refined, processed food fix will only appease a problem that will reoccur two or three hours following their last snack or meal. I sympathize with this situation. Parents march into the grocery store with the best intentions of purchasing healthy, vibrant foods for their children. Unfortunately, confusing products with claims such as, "filled with real fruit," "fortified with vitamin B," and "low in fat" lead parents to believe they are buying healthy products when in fact they are not. There are many delicious alternatives that are easily accessible and healthier for the entire family. As you will read in the next section, How to Find Healthier Carbohydrates, there are ways for a parent to take action, become informed, and exercise control over this flour frenzy.

HOW THE FUEL WORKS

In order to understand how eating refined carbohydrates is linked to the above-mentioned symptoms and health problems, let's look at the roles of glucose and insulin.

When eating a carbohydrate (simple or complex), the body converts it into glucose for metabolic fuel. Glucose has three different routes it can take:

1. It can be used in the body immediately as energy.
2. It can be stored for short-term use in the liver and muscles as glycogen.
3. It can be converted into fatty acids for long-term storage (fat storage).

The liver and muscles have only a limited amount of storage space for excess glucose. According to Barry Sears, author of *The Zone*, "In the liver, you can store only about 60–90g of carbohydrates. This is the equivalent to about two cups of cooked pasta or three typical candy bars."[3] This is not a lot of storage space, and it fills up very quickly. In times of famine or starvation, stored glycogen is extremely valuable because it can be quickly converted to glucose and used as energy. Luckily, famine and starvation are quite rare in the Western world, and a regular supply of glucose from the food we eat is usually available. Today, most of the health problems experienced in North America are a result of over-, not under-indulgence. With the exception of eating disorders such as anorexia nervosa or extreme hormonal disorders, it is very rare for a person to drain his or her glycogen stores—they are usually constantly full. Now, here is a key point: once the glycogen stores are full, excess glucose is converted by insulin to be stored as fat.

THE LINK: GLUCOSE-INSULIN AXIS

The key to eating carbohydrates properly lies in understanding the intricate relationship between blood glucose levels and insulin. Insulin is a hormone secreted from the pancreas in response to elevated blood glucose levels. One of insulin's many roles in the body is the transport of glucose into the cells. The process works like this: blood glucose levels are elevated by the ingestion of a specific food, the pancreas responds by secreting insulin, insulin opens up the gates of cells to allow glucose to be absorbed, glucose gets absorbed into the cells, and blood glucose levels are normalized. For the most part, when eating a wholesome, healthy diet, this process runs quite smoothly. However, when refined flours enter the scene, this process is disturbed. To understand why refined flours disrupt this process, it important to know that the amount of insulin secreted is different for every food. Consider the following two examples. Let's say Mary ate a wholesome, unrefined complex carbohydrate such as a healthy piece of unrefined, twelve-grain bread or a delicious salad. As we now know, the body breaks down this piece of bread or salad into glucose to utilize it as fuel. The high-fiber content in this complex carbohydrate acts as a brake, causing glucose to enter the bloodstream slowly. Once blood glucose levels are elevated, a knock is heard on the door of the pancreas, indicating it is time to secrete insulin to deal with the glucose in the blood. Because glucose entered the bloodstream slowly, a suitable amount of insulin—not too much and not too little—is secreted to facilitate the transport of glucose from the blood into the cells. With no dramatic fluctuation in blood sugar levels, Mary is provided with slow-release energy, so feeling alert, awake, and happy. She has not oversecreted insulin, and therefore does not have any excess to store as fat. In addition, she has benefited from eating a high-fiber complex carbohydrate, loaded with nutrients such as vitamins A, B, C, iron, and fiber.

Now let us look at the second example. Bob decides to grab a piece of pizza on a white flour crust for lunch. Sounds fairly common, doesn't it? The dough used to make this pizza crust has been put through the refining process, bleached and stripped of its fiber (the brake). With very little fiber, this food (in the form of glucose) enters the bloodstream hurriedly. Due to the rapid speed of entry into the bloodstream, a state of high blood sugar or hyperglycemia results. Bob's body perceives this state as a potentially threatening one, and attempts to maintain balance by oversecreting the hormone insulin. Unfortunately, too much insulin will drop Bob's blood sugar to an exceedingly low level, creating the opposite condition called hypoglycemia (low blood sugar). Hypoglycemia is associated with irritability, headaches, confusion, cravings, and cold sweats. To combat these symptoms and find relief, Bob will likely reach for more sweets and refined carbs within two or three hours in an attempt to boost his energy and curb his cravings. With his next meal, the vicious cycle will begin all over again. To make matters even worse, if this cycle continues, Bob will eventually oversecrete insulin and store the excess as fat. The exact same effect occurs in our children when they eat white breads, baked goods, and other refined goodies. In kids, the wrong carbohydrate selection can be followed by episodes of hyperactivity and then a "crash" in energy and mood—not an ideal state for them to be in at school! If your children experience moodiness, discipline problems, and lack of focus at home or in school, you should check the amount of refined flours they are consuming. Before medicating their unruly behavior, it is wise to examine and optimize their nutritional intake.

> *More than 50 percent of Canadians are overweight and at high risk for diabetes, heart attack, asthma, and cancer, and that figure could reach 80 percent by 2015.*

There are additional problems when blood sugar levels rise too quickly. Eating a diet high in refined carbs for a prolonged period can cause cells to become *insulin resistant,* meaning they no longer respond to normal amounts of secreted insulin. The pancreas, desperate to maintain blood glucose levels within a normal range, will secrete more and more insulin. Excess insulin triggers the body to respond with the signal, "Slow down or I will have to store this excess insulin as fat!" In short, excess insulin = excess fat. Farmers have known for years that the best way to fatten their cattle is to feed them low-fat, highly refined grains. Thus, it is no surprise to discover that these refined carbohydrates are having the same effect on our children. As you will discover in Chapter 8, childhood obesity is at an all-time high with over 50 percent of our children suffering unnecessarily from excess weight. Switching to higher fiber, whole grains is one of many effective ways to reverse weight gain in kids before it has the opportunity to create irreversible physical and psychological damage.

There is some debate among scientists and health care experts regarding insulin resistance. Some researchers feel that certain people are genetically more susceptible to insulin resistance, and environmental components (such as the food we eat) have little or no effect. Others believe the surge in childhood obesity is more environmentally based, brought on by poor food choices such as refined carbohydrates and sugary snacks. While I believe both to be contributors, I feel the deterioration in our food quality and food production is creating a large part of the weight problem we are currently seeing in our children. The health statistics of non-Western pediatric populations such as Japanese children (who, for the most part, consume a high-fiber, non-processed food diet) show that obesity is virtually nonexistent. It is ludicrous to think that suddenly, 50 percent of our children (obesity now affects over half the children in the United States) have become genetically predisposed to insulin resistance. The epidemic rates of childhood obesity and Type II diabetes, along with the increased consumption of refined flours, are not a coincidence—it is glaring evidence.

So the question is, how do you measure the insulin response of specific carbohydrates? One way is to look at the fiber content. Remember, fiber acts as a brake and will therefore slow the entry of certain foods into the bloodstream. The slower the food enters the bloodstream, the less dramatic the insulin surge will be. Yet most parents do not have the time to measure the amount of fiber their children are eating daily. An alternate and more accurate form of measurement is to become familiar with an easy-to-use scale called the glycemic index (GI). The glycemic index measures the rate of entry of glucose into the bloodstream, thereby providing a good indication of insulin response. For ranking purposes, this scale is divided into three categories: low, medium, and high. Food is categorized from a scale of 0 to 100, depending on its effect on blood sugar levels. On the glycemic scale, the highest measurement is for glucose and has the ranking of 100. Foods that are lowest on the glycemic index have the slowest rate of entry into the bloodstream, and therefore have the lowest insulin response. The numerical categories are:

- Low (up to 55)
- Medium (56–70)
- High (over 70)

As a general rule, all unrefined complex carbohydrates such as fruits, vegetables, whole grains, and legumes provide excellent sources of energy without creating dramatic fluctuations in glucose levels. These foods generally have a lower GI rating. Refined, sugared foods such as white bread, bagels, candy, and sugary juices have a higher glycemic index rating and create a dramatic insulin response. When making your carbohydrate selections, it is best to make most of your choices from foods lower on the glycemic index. That said, do not forget the 80–20 rule discussed in Chapter 1. Food should be enjoyable, savored, and fun. If most of your selections are from lower GI healthy foods and the remaining are from higher GI foods that are occasional treats for your family, then you are doing a great job. Enjoy!

It should also be noted that not all foods with a low GI rating (such as chocolate bars) are healthy, and not all foods having a high GI rating are unhealthy. Certain chocolate bars and other processed items have a lower GI rating because of their fat content. Fat will slow down the entry of glucose into the bloodstream, causing the GI number to be lower. The scale is an indicator of glucose/insulin response, not health. Use it as one—but not your only—tool.

When looking over the scale, you may be surprised to find certain foods—such as white potatoes, bananas, and carrots—have higher GI scores. White potatoes and white rice rank fairly high on the glycemic index with their numbers being 82 and 88 respectively. Although potatoes are loaded with some essential nutrients—such as vitamin E, calcium, iron, and vitamin C—they are not the best for weight loss because of the dramatic fluctuations they cause in blood sugar levels. When searching for a potato selection, it is better to switch to a yam or a sweet potato (ranked at 54), which have less effect on glucose and insulin levels. In terms of bananas and carrots, a parent has to weigh the nutritional benefit of these natural food sources against the higher GI rating. Although certain nutritional authors stick strictly to the glycemic index ratings for weight loss, I believe that the nutritional benefits these food sources offer far outweigh their higher glycemic index ratings. I have yet to meet a child who has become obese from eating too many bananas or carrots. For a complete list of the glycemic index, visit http://www.glycemicindex.com/

In a study of 285 boys and girls, children who consumed eleven servings per week of whole grain foods were significantly leaner and had a greater insulin sensitivity than those who consumed four servings per week.[4]

How to Find Healthier Carbohydrates

Finding healthier, whole grains is much easier than it used to be. With the plethora of health food stores and nutritional products, unrefined grainy products are fairly easy to find. Everywhere you turn, there are small and large businesses trying to make a shift toward health eating. On a recent visit to the tiny (and I mean tiny!) town where I went camping as a child, I was shocked to find a fully stocked health food store. All the stores in this town comprise a mere mile, yet you can still find healthy, wholesome foods—how wonderful! When looking for whole grains, your local health food store should be your first stop. Unprocessed grains can be purchased in bulk as flours or as pre-made breads, pastas, muffin mixes, cereals, etc. Also check your local grocery store. Many bakery sections of certain large grocery chains have begun to stock unrefined, whole or cracked breads, pastas, and cookies. As with all markets, health food products are consumer driven—the more demand they have for these products, the more available they will become, and the prices will eventually drop. If you are adventurous, try purchasing the flours in bulk and baking your own bread as a cost-saving option.

What About Whole Wheat Bread?

For most of us, determining which foods are whole and which are refined can be bewildering. Instead of turning this process into a complicated science, there are a few rules that will help you distinguish the good grains from the not-so-good grains. For starters, assume that most packaged, processed carbohydrates (aside from those found in health food stores) contain refined flours. If the product in question has a long shelf life, has words you cannot pronounce on the label, or can be rolled into a ball when eaten, you are looking at refined grains. Also, become an educated label reader. If you see the words, refined, enriched, fortified, bleached, or white, the product is no longer whole. If a vitamin or mineral has to be added back into a product in a clumsy attempt to make the food whole again, it is nutritionally void. Surprisingly, even ingredients that list made from whole wheat are typically refined, void in essential nutrients, and have a high GI rating. For the most part, people think brown sugar and brown bread are healthy. In reality, most whole wheat brown breads are made from white flour with some added bran to make the flour appear brown. Tricky, isn't it? To safeguard against this, make sure your whole wheat bread lists the words "unrefined flours" to be sure you're eating a whole grain food.

The world of healthier grains is not something you learn about overnight. Have fun experimenting and learning different ways to cook them. If you wish to delve even deeper into this subject, *Amazing Grains: Creating Main Dishes with Whole Grains* by Joanne Saltzman provides excellent recipes. The following are some grains that are higher in fiber, protein, minerals, and vitamins and have typically not been through the refining process. Please refer to the chart below for individual cooking times.

Amaranth. Amaranth can taste mild, sweet, and nutty or malt-like depending on the variety of grain used. This grain has a sticky texture, so be careful not to overcook it. Amaranth has three times the amount of fiber and five times the amount of iron content compared to wheat. It contains no gluten and is therefore suitable for people suffering from wheat allergies. Amaranth can be used in the preparation of flatbreads, pancakes, pastas, and cereals, or popped and eaten as popcorn.

Brown rice. The milling process is the difference that separates white rice from brown rice. The outer bran layer is removed from white rice, stripping away the fiber, vitamin B, and essential oils. Brown rice can be made into tasty breads and pastas, or can be used as a delicious accompaniment to a vegetable stir-fry. Because of its high-fiber content, it is no surprise that the glycemic index of brown rice is significantly lower than white rice (55 to 88 respectively).

Buckwheat. Buckwheat is an extremely popular grain in Japan where it is referred to as "the meat of fields." This grain is high in fiber, minerals, vitamins, and essential amino acids. Buckwheat also contains a bioflavonoid (a powerful antioxidant) called rutin, which improves circulation and cardiovascular health. Buckwheat can be used in noodles (called soba noodles), soups, or for biscuits.

Kamut. Kamut is an ancient relative of modern durum wheat. This grain has an extremely pleasant, rich, buttery flavor. Kamut is extremely high in protein, amino acids, lipids, vitamins, and minerals and is easily digested. Kamut is less allergenic than wheat and therefore can usually be used by those suffering from wheat allergies.

Quinoa (pronounced "keen-wa"). Quinoa is a grain that was highly revered by the ancient Incas, who called it "the mother of all grains." It has the highest protein and fat content of all the grains and is very rich in calcium and iron. Quinoa flour has a nutty flavor. This easy-to-digest grain has been receiving a lot more attention because it is wheat free and can be eaten by those who are allergic to wheat. This grain is suitable for infant cereals, rice replacements, casseroles, soups, and stews.

Millet. Millet is a mild-tasting grain that is an excellent source of minerals and vitamins such as folate, vitamin K, calcium, magnesium, phosphorus, copper, iron, and potassium. This grain is easily digestible and is beneficial for people suffering from intestinal disorders and for managing blood sugar imbalances. It is an excellent grain for bulking up various stews or chilis.

Spelt. A relative of wheat, spelt is a hearty, tasty grain, loaded with fiber, protein, and vitamin B. It is a potential option for those suffering from gluten insensitivity. Spelt is very versatile, and its flour is used to create breads, pastas, cookies, crackers, cakes, waffles, and pancakes. Spelt has a hard, protective husk that shields it from pollutants and insects, so farmers can avoid using pesticides.

Cooking Times for Grains

Grains (1 cup)	Cups of water	Approx. Cooking Time
Amaranth	1½	20 minutes
Brown rice	2	45–60 minutes
Buckwheat	2	15 minutes
Kamut	1	60 minutes
Millet	3	40–45 minutes
Quinoa	2	15 minutes
Spelt	2½–3	2 hours +

Source: http://www.thebigcarrot.ca/cookinggrains.htm

"I realized making the switch to healthier grains was easier than I thought. I give my kids kamut pasta, cereal, and pack their lunches with spelt bread! My son is even eating macaroni and cheese with whole-grain rice pasta! As for baking, I have switched my flours to the healthier flours for cookies and other recipes."
—BUNNY DENTON, Oakville, Ontario

Although healthier grain selections are always the best choice for kids, they are not always readily available. Sleepovers, school trips, birthday parties, and vacations make it very difficult to always serve the highest quality grains to your children. With children's busy schedules, healthy nutrition may fall by the wayside. The important thing is to ensure that most of their grains are derived from wholesome sources. Stocking your cupboards with healthier grains in the form of cereals, cookies, breads, and pastas will ensure that they will be the staples eaten at home. Consider the following tricks of the trade to incorporate hearty, healthy, grainy products in your children's lives:

Instead of:	Switch to:
A sandwich on white or whole wheat bread	Kamut, spelt, or twelve-grain bread
White or whole wheat spaghetti with tomato sauce	Spelt pasta with fresh vegetables and tomato sauce
Packaged, refined cookies	Homemade carob chip cookies baked with spelt flour
Sugary, fortified cereals	Oatmeal, kamut or quinoa cereal, naturally sweetened
White hot dog or hamburger buns	Multigrain or brown rice buns

HEALTHIER TREATS

Looking for healthier treats but don't know where to start? This healthy chocolate chip recipe is a real winner for the kids in my family. Try it as a first step to getting acquainted with healthier grains.

Scrumptious Spelt Oatmeal Chocolate Chip Cookies

YIELDS 3 DOZEN

1 cup olive oil
1 cup maple syrup
1 tsp vanilla
¼ cup boiling water
1 cup spelt whole flour *(available in bulk form in health food* *stores or some grocery stores)*
1 tsp salt
1 tsp baking soda
2 cups oatmeal
¼ cup flaxseeds or ½ cup flaked coconut
1 cup chocolate chips

Beat oil, maple syrup, and vanilla with beater for 2 minutes until foamy. Add boiling water and stir. Add flour, salt, baking soda, and oatmeal and stir with wooden spoon. Mix in flaxseeds or coconut and chocolate chips. On nonstick or lightly greased cookie sheet, flatten out small balls of dough with fork. Bake at 325°F for 18–25 minutes.

Parents often feel slightly tense about introducing any sort of new food into their children's diet. Fearful of a family protest or worried that their children may go hungry, some feel it would be easier to stick with what they know. Of course it would be easier—not healthier, but easier. And really, what is more important? Depending on your children's disposition, taste buds, and moods on that particular day, it's possible that they might refuse dinner now and then, but don't worry. Children do not go hungry for long and will eventually eat what they are served and learn what is healthy. You will be surprised to see that with patience and persistence, your kids will start to accept and even enjoy new, healthier selections. In addition, you will feel an enormous sense of satisfaction knowing that you have just provided your family with nourishing, vibrant food. Getting your kids and the entire family into the habit of eating wholesome grains is a major step toward greater health and wellness.

There are two routes you can take when introducing a new food into your children's diet. There is the "sneak it in and hope they don't notice" approach or the "educate and participate" approach. From my experience in dealing with young tummies, kids are smart and *they can't be fooled!* Children as young as one or two are aware of new foods being introduced into their diet. However, if you have found that sneaking in healthy foods is the only way to get it onto your children's plates and into their stomachs, go for it. If this approach does not work, you may want to consider the "educate and participate" approach. Often it is to a parent's advantage to set up a bond of trust so their children can feel free to express opinions about what foods they like or dislike. The educate and participate approach teaches children the fundamentals of healthy eating, while allowing them to exercise some control over their individual food choices. If your children are old enough to understand the health benefits of specific foods, explain it to them. The more they understand about food and nutrition, the more likely they will continue healthy eating patterns in the future. Provide children with explanations that relate to their value systems such as, "You will be able to play soccer with more energy," or "This food helps to protect you from getting sick." Children are very fast learners and are usually more in touch with their bodies than most adults. The educate and participate approach allows your children to take an active role in their food selections, while giving their little voices the attention they deserve. Invite your children along to discover and experiment with the new world of grains. Have them help you prepare cookies or bake bread with these new options. Getting them familiar with health food stores or health food sections will open their eyes to new, nutritional treats for them to munch on!

People of Okinawa, a Japanese island, are the longest-living people in the world and are considered youngsters at ages seventy, eighty, and ninety. Their low levels of hormone-dependent cancers, Type II diabetes, and obesity have been linked to their high intake of complex carbohydrates and whole grains.[5]

PHYTONUTRIENTS: WHAT ARE THEY AND WHERE CAN I GET THEM?

The amount of fresh fruits and vegetables eaten by children today is alarmingly low. Healthy after-school snacks such as fresh apple slices, juicy oranges, and raw carrots and celery sticks have been replaced with sugary fruit roll-ups, chips, and big-gulp slurpies. Sadly, North American children frequently fail to meet the daily national dietary recommendations of fruits and vegetables. In one study, it was found that the average American child consumed only one serving of fruits or vegetables per day.[6] That is a far cry from the three to five selections recommended for optimal daily health. Most national standards recommend that children between the ages of two and nineteen consume approximately three to five servings of vegetables per day

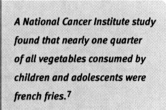

A National Cancer Institute study found that nearly one quarter of all vegetables consumed by children and adolescents were french fries.[7]

and two to four fruits. These amounts may vary depending on each child's age, weight, and physical activity. When providing your children with fruit and vegetables, try to select mostly from whole, fresh, live produce instead of sugary fruit drinks or canned selections.

What comprises a serving? According to the Food Guide Pyramid for Young Children, servings for vegetables and fruits are:

Vegetables
- ½ cup of chopped raw or cooked vegetables
- 1 cup of raw leafy vegetables

Fruits
- 1 piece of fruit or melon wedge
- ¾ cup of juice
- ½ cup of canned fruit
- ½ cup of dried fruit

It is no great secret that fruits and vegetables are loaded with essential vitamins, minerals, and fiber; however, recent scientific advancements have enabled researchers to identify additional chemical components called *phytonutrients*. Phytonutrients can be found in fruits, vegetables, soy products, and whole grains. These chemicals play a role in disease prevention. Unlike vitamins or minerals, a lack of phytonutrients does not appear to create a deficiency. Still, these powerful components offer very potent protection against certain diseases. According to the American Dietetic Association, phytonutrients are associated with the prevention of and/or treatment of the four leading causes of death in the United States: cancer, diabetes, cardiovascular disease, and hypertension.[8] We are just beginning to understand the role that phytonutrients play in disease prevention, and researchers are discovering new ones every day. To date, over 900 phytonutrients have been discovered. There are an estimated 100 different phytonutrients available in each serving of vegetables.[9] The health benefits and future nutritional insurance provided by phytonutrients are immeasurable, which is another reason to fill up your family's plates with fruits and veggies!

The following are examples of some of the most widely known and researched phytonutrients:

Phytonutrients: Their Sources and Benefits

Name	Food Sources	Health Benefits
CAROTENOIDS		
Examples: Lutein, lycopene, beta-carotene	Bright yellow, orange, and red plant pigments (tomatoes, yams, squash, berries, and plums)	Offer protection against certain cancers such as breast, uterine, and prostate
FLAVONOIDS		
Examples: Quercitin, rutin, hesperidin	Citrus fruits, grapefruit, and buckwheat	Provide protection against allergies, inflammation, and free radical damage
ISOFLAVONES		
Examples: Genistein, daidzein	Soy products and other beans and legumes	Block enzymes that promote tumor growth
ALLYLIC SULFIDES		
Examples: Part of thiol subclass	Garlic and onions (need to be mashed for benefits to be achieved)	Are natural antifungal, anti-bacterial, and anti-parasite; boost immune system

Leafy green and cruciferous vegetables such as broccoli, cauliflower, cabbage, spinach, bok choy, kale, and Brussels sprouts are also loaded with a hearty mix of various phytonutrients.

Now, here is the challenge. How can you slowly introduce vibrant, healthy foods into your children's daily diet without a fuss? Consider the following tips:

- Keep cut-up fruits and vegetables in the house with tasty, healthy dips such as hummus (chickpea dip), natural peanut butter, or salsa.

  Broccoli and broccoli sprouts contain a chemical called sulfurophane, which kills the bacteria helicobacter pylori, responsible for stomach ulcers and most stomach cancers.

- Offer your children a variety of fruits and/ or vegetables. This allows them to exercise their independence over their eating likes and dislikes.

- Replace snack foods such as sugary fruit roll-ups or a juice box with the real thing— fruit!

- Make sure every meal has at least one live, raw fruit or vegetable on your child's plate.

- Urge your kids to chew their fruits and vegetables slowly and completely. Chewing food breaks down the vital nutrients into absorbable, digestible units.

  Lower levels of the type of nutrients found in fruits and vegetables are associated with poor academic performance. Supplementation can improve cognitive abilities in children by raising blood nutrient concentrations.

- Make your children's plates look like a box of Crayola crayons! Including a variety of colors on their plates will ensure they are receiving a cross-spectrum of nutrients.

- For a treat, try chocolate-dipped fruit instead of refined, processed chocolate chip cookies.

The younger the children are when they are introduced to fresh fruits and vegetables, the more likely they will be to accept and ask for them as part of their meals.

MAKING LIFE EASIER FOR PARENTS

Because of busy schedules and the reality that parents can't always get children to eat as many fruits and veggies as they should, I recommend purchasing a fortifier that can be mixed into a child's drink in the morning. That way parents can breathe a little bit easier knowing their children are receiving an extra boost of greens. Fortifiers, such as green powders designed for kids, should not be used to replace healthy eating; rather, they should be considered as an excellent nutritional safety net.

I highly recommend the product called greens+ kids, which can be purchased at most health food stores. One serving supplies a child with a hearty serving of disease-fighting phytochemicals. The product is certified organic and contains a mixture of over twenty-five fruits and vegetables, plant nutrients, and non-dairy bacterial cultures for immune system and gastrointestinal health and brain-boosting elements. It has a natural berry taste and a purple color that turns water into a fun shade, or can be disguised in juice. Allow your children to do the mixing so they can participate in healthy living activities.

IS ORGANIC REALLY NECESSARY?

When shopping for fruits and veggies, produce labeled "certified organic" is always best. Most of the produce in our supermarkets have been heavily sprayed with herbicides and pesticides and have a waxy, shiny finish, making them appear "pretty" to consumers. We have to step back and think—we wouldn't feed our dog wax or harmful pesticides, so why are we letting our children eat them? As you discovered in Chapter 2, it is far too early to know what kinds of health consequences herbicides, pesticides, and other toxins will have on future generations. According to Leading Edge International Research Group:

> *There is abundant evidence of the risk that toxic pesticides pose to human health. The most vulnerable populations are children, the developing fetus, the elderly, the ill and immunocompromised, and those with asthma, allergies and other medical conditions. Most worrisome from a public health perspective are chronic health effects*

such as cancer, infertility, miscarriage, birth defects, and effects on the brain and nervous system.[10]

The environmental costs of spraying with pesticides and herbicides are another issue to consider. Pesticide and herbicide usage is wreaking havoc on our soil, air, fish, and other wildlife. This issue may feel too large to tackle—that switching your family to organic foods would not make much difference in the larger scheme of things. Trust me, it will. Slowly but surely, more and more people are recognizing the environmental problems created by various food manufacturing practices. The public want to know more about the effects foods have on the quality of their families' lives and on the earth. Taking small steps toward health, whether it is buying certified organic produce or making healthy snacks available for your children, can have immeasurable positive health benefits. If money allows, switch to organic. Check out local organic farmers and markets. It is often cheaper to buy from them than from the grocery or health food stores. Organic produce usually does not look as colorful and shiny as non-organic produce. Remember, nature did not design fruits and vegetables to look this way—we did. Big and beautiful, waxy and perfect does not necessarily mean nutritious and safe. If organic is too costly, I recommend purchasing a potato scrubber and natural produce soap from your local health food store to vigorously wash your fruits and veggies prior to eating. This process removes some, not all, of the toxins.

TRY

1. **Having your children eat fruit and drink water! Drinking boxes are filled with refined carbs and sugars that will do your children no good! Provide them with clean drinking water for liquid and fresh fruit for snacks.**

   ■

2. **Avoiding products with the following words listed in the ingredients: "bleached," "fortified," "refined," or "enriched" flour.**

■

3. Using whole grain flours for cooking or baking such as spelt, buckwheat, quinoa, amaranth, and brown rice. These flours are available in all forms in most health food stores and some grocery stores, and can be purchased as pastas, breads, muffin mixes, and cereals.

■

4. Eliminating fast foods. These foods have large quantities of refined carbohydrates.

■

5. Avoiding grain products that are labeled "low fat." Most of these products use refined grains and are loaded with sugar to compensate for taste. Remember, these products typically promote, not prevent, weight gain.

NOTES

1 A. Weil, *Eating Well for Optimum Health* (New York: Alfred A. Knopf, 2000).

2 C. Bateson-Koch, *Allergies—Disease in Disguise* (Burnaby, BC: Alive Books, 1994).

3 B. Sears, *The Zone* (New York: ReganBooks, 1995).

4 *The Medical Post*, "Nutrition" (December 18, 2001).

5 B. Wilcox, C. Wilcox, and M. Suzuki, *The Okinawa Program* (New York: Clarkson Potter Publishers, 2001).

6 W. Craig, "Phytochemicals: Guardians of Our Health," *JADA* 97(10): S199–S204.

7 www.cspinet.org.

8 A. Bloch et al., "Position of the American Dietetic Association: Phytochemicals and Functional Foods," *JADA* 95:493–496.

9 M. Polk, "Feast on Phytochemicals," AICR newsletter Issue 51.

10 Leading Edge International Research Group, About Pesticides, www.igc.apc.org.

CHAPTER 5

Protein Power for Kids

PROTEINS ARE THE second category of macronutrients that are a necessary part of every child's diet. The building blocks of protein are called *amino acids*. There are twenty-two amino acids in total; nine are classified as *essential*, meaning the body cannot synthesize them, so they must come from the diet. The remaining thirteen are *non-essential*, meaning the body can synthesize them and they do not have to be derived from food sources. Proteins serve many functions in the body, such as maintaining proper growth and repair of muscles and tissues; manufacturing hormones, antibodies, and enzymes; and preserving the proper acid-alkali balance in the body.

Proteins are classified into two categories: complete and incomplete. Complete proteins contain all the essential amino acids and are found primarily in animal sources such as meat, poultry, fish, eggs, and dairy products. Incomplete proteins do not have at least one of the essential amino acids and are found in fruits, vegetables, grains, and legumes. It was once thought that vegetarians, who consume mostly incomplete proteins, achieved proper amounts of protein only by carefully combining incomplete proteins at one meal. For example, combinations of incomplete proteins to form complete proteins are:

- Rice and beans
- Cereal and milk
- Beans and corn
- Bread and cheese

Current research demonstrates that such tedious combinations are no longer necessary. We now know that incomplete proteins can be stored in the body for many days and can be combined with other incomplete proteins long after a meal is consumed to form complete ones. This is good news for vegetarians, who were frustrated by fussing with measurements and proper combinations at every meal or snack. If a wide variety of incomplete proteins are consumed over a day or two, the body can balance the various amino acids properly to form and preserve the necessary muscles and body tissue.

The average American consumes about 100 grams of protein a day, primarily from animal sources.

Similar to carbohydrates, 1 gram of protein yields 4 calories. Children require approximately 20–25 percent of their total daily caloric intake from protein. The truth is that most North American kids today eat about twice as much protein as they need. It is easy to figure out how much protein a child requires. Simply multiply the amount of calories a child eats daily by 20–25% and then divide by 4 for the calorie yield of proteins. For example, if a child consumes 1800 calories per day the equation would be; 1800 (calories) x 0.20 (20%) divided by 4 = 90 grams of protein

Let's have a look at some common foods and their protein sources in grams:

Amounts of Protein in Food Sources

Food Source	Protein in Grams
Chicken, baked, 3 oz	28
Sirloin steak, 3 oz	25
Salmon, 3 oz	22
Cow's milk, 1 cup	8
Egg, 1 large	6
Soybeans, 1 cup	29
Veggie burger, 1 patty	5–24
Lima beans, 1 cup	15
Peanut butter, 2 tbsp	8
Brown rice, 1 cup	5
Broccoli, cooked, 1cup	5
Cashews, ¼ cup	2.7

Source: www.vrg.org/nutrition/protein.htm

WHAT ABOUT MEAT?

The million-dollar question parents want answered is, "Do my children need meat to grow healthy and strong?" Many still believe that animal products are superior in the amount and type of protein they provide. There is a perception that meat = protein = strength and health for children. While it is true that meat can provide a good source of protein, parents should be aware of all the information in order to make an informed choice they feel comfortable with. Keep these ideas in mind:

- Health hazards for children have been linked to the consumption and production of certain meats.

- Healthier substitutions that provide excellent and equivalent sources of protein are now widely available and are kid-friendly too.

Nitrates

Among children's favorite protein selections, foods such as hot dogs, luncheon meats (bologna), and hamburgers rank quite high. A 1996 poll sponsored by the National Hot Dog and Sausage Council showed that 37 percent of parents reported that their children requested hot dogs as their first choice at warm weather events and 27 percent reported hamburgers as their second choice.[1] One of the concerns with the consumption of certain meats such as hot dogs has to do with the usage of preservatives called nitrates. Nitrates are added to hot dogs, bacon, ham, bologna, and sausages to help meat keep its red, pinkish colour. Without the nitrates, the meat would turn gray. When nitrates combine with gastric juices in the stomach, a dangerous compound called nitrosamine is formed. Nitrosamine has been found to be carcinogenic (cancer causing) when tested on most laboratory animals. In addition, nitrates bind to hemoglobin, which blocks it from carrying life-sustaining oxygen. High levels of nitrates can cause "blue baby syndrome," a condition in which an infant turns blue due to a lack of oxygen in the system.[2] Other symptoms of nitrate toxicity include hyperactivity, dizziness, and

> *Children who ate hot dogs once a week doubled their chances of brain tumors; those who ate them twice a week tripled it.*[3]

vomiting. Due to this known toxic effect, nitrates are banned from baby foods. If it is unsafe for infant food, shouldn't it be unsafe for all humans to consume? However, the ability of nitrates to reduce the chance of botulism poisoning is one reason why they are used in our food. Nitrate-free meats are now available at some health food stores and butchers. Luckily, there are many meat-free substitutes for the standard hot dogs and/or luncheon meats, eliminating the entire nitrate problem. Please refer to Appendix I for a list of delicious alternative meat products that can provide the entire family with healthy, safe, nitrate-free options.

The Health of Our Animals—or Lack of It

Aside from the moral question of how we are currently treating animals (that I leave up to the individual reader to decide), people need to know how the health status of our animals is silently taking its toll on the health of our children.

A major concern and controversy with meat consumption is the amount and type of medications fed to or injected into animals prior to their slaughter. Drugs such as antibiotics and hormones are routinely given to livestock without the public's awareness or consent. The use of antibiotics is to ensure animals are infection free. Unfortunately, the conditions in slaughterhouses are appalling and unsanitary. To a cattle farmer, an animal with a cold or respiratory infection is a potential financial loss. To prevent a few infectious animals from tainting the entire herd, antibiotics are commonly added to the food fed to all the livestock. The danger of this practice is that residues of these medications end up in the food we serve our families. A recent article in TIME exposed an unsettling case, documenting the course of action taken by a farmer when chickens developed signs of an infection:

> A respiratory infection, if that's what they have, could spread to the 20,000 other birds in the chicken house in a matter of days. The vet recommends the antibiotic enrofloxacin—the animal version of Cipro. Since it's not practical to treat the birds individually, the farmer pours a 5-g jug of the drug into the flock's drinking water.[4]

The article went on to state that 80 percent of all the antibiotics used in the United States are used for agricultural purposes. Scary isn't it?

The truth is, we are unsure of how the abuse of antibiotics will affect the future health of our children. We do know two things: that antibiotic usage is greater than ever before and that antibiotic resistance is on the rise. Coincidence? It is virtually impossible to say for sure, but it is a fact that must be considered. Science continues to chase bugs with drugs, only to discover smarter, more powerful bugs. With bacteria's ability to adapt and mutate faster than the pace of medical research, microorganisms are winning the race. Careful consideration and proper steps need to be taken to reduce the amount of antibiotics and other medications put into animals' feed. Raising animals in more humane environments is one of many steps that can be taken. If you are interested in reading more about the method of meat and dairy production in North America, *Diet for a New America*, by John Robbins, is an excellent resource to have in your home library.

Heart Healthy

The last concern with meat consumption is its fat content. Red meats such as hamburgers, steak, ribs, etc., and dairy products contain a large amount of saturated fat. An overconsumption of saturated fat will raise blood cholesterol, clog arteries, and make your child's heart work harder than it should. With obesity and Type II diabetes occurring at epidemic rates in our young, red meat is not recommended as a daily staple. Switching to fish and/or poultry is one very effective step that will help reduce the amount of saturated fat in your child's system. Cold-water fish (such as tuna, salmon, and halibut) are excellent sources of protein for kids and are packed with powerful omega-3 fatty acids, which are necessary for proper brain development. Other excellent alternative sources of protein are whole grains, nuts, soy, and legumes.

Children on the typical North American diet get approximately 70% of their protein from animal sources. Children in China and vegetarians, in contrast, get approximately 90 percent of their protein from vegetable sources. There is an enormous difference in the heart disease risk of these two groups. For example, coronary heart disease is present to some degree, (often undetected), in at least 70 percent of American adults, but only 3 percent of those from rural China who consume a vegetarian-based diet suffer from heart disease.

THE JOY OF SOY

For some strange reason, the words soy, tofu, tempeh, or textured vegetable protein seem to scare people a bit. Soy protein is often associated with tasteless, slippery white cubes that children wouldn't dare eat. As a dedicated vegetarian who has enjoyed soy for years, I can only guess that the misunderstanding of this humble bean and its by-products is due to lack of familiarity. In truth, there is a lot more to soy than just blocks of bland tofu. Ice cream, veggie burgers, miso soup, pie filling, hot dogs— you name it— are all available.

Not only is soy delicious, it has also been receiving many nutritional accolades as well. In fact, the US Food and Drug Administration (FDA) has authorized the use of a health claim linking the consumption of soy products to a reduction in coronary heart disease. The FDA's claim was approved after reviewing more than twenty years of scientific research on the benefits of soy. According to the FDA, 25 grams of soy per day helps reduce the risk of the development of coronary heart disease. This is significant news for the millions of North Americans suffering from plaque buildup in their arteries, high blood pressure, or for those who have a history of heart disease. In fact, this news is not only significant for adults, it is also pertinent information for our youth. As mentioned, doctors and researchers are now finding arterial constriction and plaque buildup in the arteries of children as young as five years. Arterial plaque does not occur overnight. The clogging of arteries slowly and silently occurs at any age due to faulty food choices and lack of exercise. Eating "heart healthy" food such as soy at a young age will have long-term health benefits for the future state of your child's arteries.

> *"Nothing will benefit human health and increase chances for survival of life on earth as much as the evolution to a vegetarian diet."*
> —ALBERT EINSTEIN

Further research on soy has also demonstrated that this protein source is packed with cancer-fighting phytonutrients necessary for disease prevention. One group of phytonutrients, known to be plentiful in soy, are *phytoestrogens*. According to the researchers of the book *The Okinawa Program*, "They [soy products] provide a weak form of estrogen where the body needs it and block the body's own estrogen in locations where estrogen may induce cancer."[5] In other words, eating one selection of soy per day appears to balance out the body's estrogen levels. It is thought that the Okinawans' (a group of Japanese who have the greatest amount of centenarians than any other group) high intake of soy products is partially responsible for their low rates of breast, prostate, and ovarian cancer. Soy products are also low in saturated fat, rich in omega-3 essential fatty acids (the good fat), and are an excellent source of calcium, iron, zinc, and the B vitamins.

So, how do you find soy products in a delicious, palatable form for you and your kids? With so many innovative soy derivatives, it is no longer difficult to find tasty alternatives to meat. In fact, even some fast-food chains such as McDonald's are now offering a veggie burger as a healthier option for their customers. This is one giant leap for the international fast-food industry and evidence that consumer demand for healthier products is being met. If you are looking for yummy, delicious meat alternatives to try at home, I recommend the imitation meat products available in the produce section of most grocery stores. Most of these products are made from soy protein and are free of cholesterol, preservatives, and fat. They are available as hot dogs, hamburgers, pepperoni, bologna, ground beef (perfect for chili or nachos), etc. Their taste and texture are similar to meat and they are easy to use. Try a pepperoni pizza or veggie ground beef on nacho chips (my personal favorites) with your children. They will love it!

About 90 percent of the world's soy products are genetically modified. As mentioned, it is far too early to know if there are any health implications with the genetic modification of foods. Soy products labeled non-GMO have not been genetically modified.

As will be discussed in the chapter on allergies, some children may be sensitive or allergic to soy. I do not recommend serving too many soy selections. Having soy for three meals a day is not a good idea. Eating too much soy can cause a child's body to eventually start rejecting it. One selection of soy per day is plenty. Examples of soy selections for your children are:

- One 8 ounce glass of soy milk
- 1 cup of flavored soybeans
- One container of soy yogurt
- One veggie burger
- 1 cup of edamame

Some Soy Savvy Ideas

- Include silken tofu (soft tofu) in a morning milkshake to make it creamier.

- Investigate tofu/soy cheeses, such as cream cheese, cheese slices, and shredded cheeses. (See Appendix I for delicious options.)

- Keep flavored soy nuts as snacks for your kids. Soy nuts are available in salt and vinegar, barbeque, and honey roasted flavors.

- Purchase very firm tofu, cut it into cubes, and marinate. Stir-fry as you would meat. The firmer the tofu, the higher the protein content.

- Try edamame! Eat it as a snack instead of popcorn! Edamame are the actual soybeans and are a favorite treat in Japan. Boil for five minutes, add salt or pepper, and remove the skin. Pinch the side of the pods and the beans will pop directly into your mouth. Edamame is now found in the frozen food section at most health food stores or in some Japanese shops. (One cup of edamame contains: 30 percent of a day's fiber, 20 percent of a day's vitamin C, 10 percent of a day's vitamin A, 16 grams of protein, and 200 calories.)[6]

> *Soy products are an excellent source of protein! One ½ cup of cooked soybeans is equal to 1 ounce of meat.*

Here is a recipe to enjoy with your family.

Delicious and Healthy Nachos

SERVES 2–3

1 onion, diced

1 green pepper, diced

2 Tbsp. olive oil

1 package veggie ground beef

1 cup salsa (mild, medium, or hot)

1 bag baked nacho chips

soy or low-fat shredded cheese to taste

Sauté onion and green pepper in olive oil over medium heat for 5 minutes. Add veggie ground beef and salsa into skillet. Stir and let simmer for 5 minutes.

Spread baked nacho chips on a foil-covered cookie sheet. Spread ground beef mixture over the nachos. Sprinkle with shredded cheese. Bake at 350°F for 10 minutes and enjoy!

The key with soy is to experiment. If you find a product you do not like, try others. Luckily, there are a multitude of options to select from.

If you want to include a minimal amount of red meat or chicken in your child's diet but are concerned about hormones and antibiotics, inquire about organic meats at your local butcher, or visit your local health food store or farmers' market in your area.

MILK: DOES IT DO THE BODY GOOD?

Recently, I was a guest on a call-in radio show discussing alternatives to dairy products for allergic and asthmatic children. As the show progressed, a fairly heated debate ensued. I soon realized that there were two distinct opinions about milk and its necessity as part of a child's healthy diet. Half of the callers phoned in to say that when milk and dairy products were eliminated from their children's diet, various problems, including chronic ear infections, colic, eczema, and asthma, disappeared. As I am familiar with allergic reactions to milk and have seen many cases of it in my practice, I was not surprised. The other half of the callers were parents who thought milk and dairy were essential for proper bone development, and expressed concern about finding another source of calcium. Sounds fairly reasonable doesn't it? We have all grown up with the same milk mantra—that milk does the body good—or does it? In fact, a number of callers were ardently defending milk's reputation as the most perfect food on earth and thought the link between milk and illnesses was pure quackery!

So, where does the truth lie? In the field of nutrition, there are no absolutes. Every child is biochemically different, and no one food or diet is appropriate in every situation. Health care professionals are similar to private investigators—they search for the evidence or clues that lead to the development of various illnesses or symptoms in the body. In terms of milk, the evidence is abundantly clear. Research has demonstrated that milk, once thought of as white liquid gold, is the number one food allergen for children. This fact begs the question: are we drinking milk because it is healthy, or because it is what we have always been taught to do?

According to Michael Klaper, MD, and author of *Pregnancy, Children and the Vegan Diet*:

> *Humans are the only creatures that drink milk from the mother of another species. It's as unnatural for a child to drink the milk of a cow as it is for a dog to nurse from a giraffe! Human children have no nutritional requirements for cow's milk and grow up healthy and strong without it. Cow's milk and the products made from it are laced with foreign, frequently allergy-inciting bovine protein and often contain hydrocarbon pesticides and other chemical contaminants, as well as health-endangering saturated fat. Clinical experience suggests that cow's milk is linked to numerous common health problems (runny noses, allergies, ear infections, recurrent bronchitis, asthma, etc.) that often keep people returning to their doctor's offices instead of to their jobs or classrooms. Parents should feel good about giving their children the many nutritious, tasty alternatives to dairy product instead.[7]*

Cow's milk consumption has been linked to various health problems in children that include:

- Allergic rhinitis (runny nose)
- Allergic shiners (dark circles under eyes)
- Bed-wetting
- Ear infections
- Chest infections
- Constipation
- Frequent crying
- Heart disease
- Juvenile diabetes (Type I diabetes)
- Spitting up
- Stomach aches

Breast Milk

Of course, in a baby's first year, breast milk is always best for several reasons. Breast milk is filled with essential enzymes that assist a baby's immature digestive system in digesting and absorbing its first form of food. A mother's milk also jump-starts a baby's immune system by providing the infant with protective antibodies called immunoglobins. Studies show that children who are breast-fed suffer less from allergies, ear infections, rashes, and diarrhea, and have lower rates of hospital admissions. In nature's innate wisdom, breast milk (similar to cow's milk for calves) is considered *species specific*, meaning it is designed perfectly to meet the nutritional needs of a particular species. When examining the history of milk consumption, humans are the only species that regularly consumes the milk of another. Some feel that drinking the milk of another species is unnatural and may be responsible for various health problems in our children. Consider the many differences between a cow's anatomy and a human's. Cows have four stomachs and double their body weight within forty-seven days. Human babies have only one stomach and take approximately 180 days to double their body weight. There is also considerably more protein in cow's milk than in human milk. Cow's milk derives 15 percent of its calories from protein, whereas in human milk it's 5 percent.[8] In Chapter 10 on allergies, I will show it is the undigested protein molecules, (particularly *casein*) that create allergic responses in children, leading to inflammation, asthma, eczema, and other digestive problems. Infant formulas definitely lag far behind breast milk in providing a foundation for optimal immunity. Because cow's milk and dairy formulas are pasteurized, most of the essential enzymes necessary for proper digestion are destroyed by the time they make it into a formula. Without these enzymes, digestion of the unfamiliar proteins in formula becomes extremely taxing on a baby's tiny system.

In addition to being enzyme deficient, most dairy and non-dairy formulas are also deficient in omega-3 essential fatty acids, which are necessary for proper brain, nerve, and cellular development. If formula feeding is necessary, I recommend supplementing with a good quality brand of omega-3 oil. One or two capsules can be broken up and put into a bottle, or ½–1 teaspoon of high-quality flaxseed oil or fish oil can be added. Many fish oils are now available in palatable "kid friendly" forms.

The State of Health of Our Cows

Similar to meat, the amount of antibiotics and hormones in milk and dairy products is of great concern. In the United States, it is standard practice for growth hormones to be injected into cows to make them more efficient milk producers. In her book, *Total Health Makeover,* author Marilu Henner cites:

> In the mid 1800s, the average cow yielded just under two quarts of milk per day. By 1960, the yield was over just nine quarts per day. Today, cows can yield up to fifty quarts of milk a day. That's an average of 18,000 pounds of milk per cow, per year.[9]

We are definitely pushing our cows to an unnatural limit that is taking a tremendous toll on their health and ours. The specific hormone used in the United States that has received a tremendous amount of negative publicity is called recombinant bovine growth hormone (rBGH), produced by Monsanto and sold by the trade name Posilac. The US Food and Drug Administration approved the use of this genetically engineered hormone in 1993, declaring it "safe for human consumption." At this time, Canada, Australia, and the entire European Union have banned the use of this controversial hormone. Currently in the United States, thousands of animals are injected with rBGH, which eventually reaches the public through most dairy products such as milk, cheese, yogurt, and ice cream. Upon closer inspection of the approval of the usage of the bovine growth hormone, it appears that major gaps may have occurred in the preliminary studies examining its safety and side effects. Recent research indicates that rBGH is not safe for human consumption and causes an increase in the level of a hormone called insulin growth hormone (IGF-1). Elevated levels of IGF-1 are thought to increase cell proliferation, resulting in the development of breast, prostate, and colon cancer.[10]

While the development of cancer in your children is a remote possibility, it is still wise to take every precaution when it comes to their health. It is important to realize that cancer is a multistep process—it does not develop overnight. By definition, cancer is an alteration in the architecture of our cells, creating a situation of complete cellular disorganization. In other words, our cells lose control. In terms of the hormone Posilac injected into cattle, we can only speculate and hope that it does not create detrimental health problems in our children. To date, the research on it does not look good. Unfortunately, labels on dairy products do not indicate whether they come from cows injected with this or other hormones. Who would buy them? In the United States and in Canada, to avoid unwanted hormones or antibiotics, the best safety measure is to purchase organic milk and milk products that are labeled free of antibiotics and hormones. Consider it as part of the "cost" of raising your children into the healthy adults they were meant to be.

Lactose Intolerance

"I'll have a decaf, double cappuccino with lactose-free milk please." Sounds like the typical order you hear at your local coffee house, doesn't it? Lactose intolerance is a problem that affects many people. In fact, 75 percent of the world's population lose the enzyme lactase after weaning. The condition of lactose intolerance commonly results in uncomfortable gastrointestinal symptoms such as bloating, cramps, flatulence, and diarrhea. The effect is caused by a shortage of the lactase enzyme, which is needed to break down lactose (milk sugar) into its simpler forms, glucose and galactose. It was once thought that people who were deficient in this enzyme were lactose intolerant. Today, the term lactose intolerance is rarely used because of the prevalence of the condition. Doctors are now using the term lactase persistence for the few people who actually retain the enzyme lactase and the ability to break down milk properly.

Where Will They Get Their Calcium?

While discussing dairy consumption, let us deal directly with the calcium issue. When I recommend eliminating milk from a child's diet, parents often ask, "Where will they get their calcium from?" To most, the notion of drinking milk for strong, healthy bones is a belief they have grown up with and trusted. A cold, white glass of milk has been equated with virtuous attributes that parents desire for their children such as health, vitality, strength, and strong bones. In terms of calcium absorption, research clearly demonstrates that milk appears to promote, not prevent, calcium loss from the bones. How does this occur? Animal and dairy products are acid-forming foods. In other words, when these foods are broken down in the body, they create an acidic residue. The body's chemistry does not like an overly acidic environment, and will make every attempt to balance this state of acidosis by using alkaline (the opposite of acid) materials as a buffer. The most abundant alkaline mineral in our body is calcium. Calcium is leached out directly from the bones in order to buffer the acidic state created by overconsumption of meat and dairy products, sugar, and refined carbohydrates. This process leads to calcium excretion through the urine. Thus, it is no surprise to find that countries with the highest consumption of dairy products, such as North America and the Scandinavian countries, also suffer from the highest levels of osteoporosis (a debilitating disease where calcium is lost directly from the bone matrix). One of the largest investigations conducted on dairy intake was a very prominent twelve-year Harvard study of 78,000 women. The results showed that those who drank milk three times a day actually broke more bones than women who rarely drank milk.[11] A similar study in Australia investigating elderly men and women found that higher dairy consumption was associated with an increased risk of fracture. Those with the highest dairy consumption had approximately twice the risk of hip fracture when compared to those with the lowest intake of dairy.[12] Other factors that promote calcium excretion from the bones are sugar consumption, smoking, a deficiency of vitamin D, and soft drinks.

ALTERNATIVE CALCIUM SOURCES

If we turn to nature, it is evident that other hearty sources of calcium-rich foods are readily available and highly absorbable. For example, leafy greens such as broccoli, kale, and collards contain an absorption rate of calcium greater than 50 percent, while milk's absorption rate is only 32 percent. Some other kid-friendly, dairy-free sources include calcium-fortified soy milk and dairy-free soy imitation products such as ice cream, cheeses, milks, yogurts, and sour cream. Calcium-fortified orange juice, nuts and seeds, salmon, and whole grain products also contain excellent levels of highly absorbable calcium. The daily calcium requirement recommended for children ages four to eight is 800 milligrams and 1,300 milligrams for ages nine to eighteen. Consider the following examples:

Milligrams of Calcium in Selected Dairy Products

- 8-ounce glass of non-fat milk = 290–300 milligrams
- 1 ounce of cheese = 130–200 milligrams
- 4 ounces of cottage cheese = 100 milligrams
- 1 tablespoon of Parmesan cheese = 69 milligrams

Milligrams of Calcium in Non-dairy Food Sources

- 1 cup of sesame seeds = 2,200 milligrams
- 1 cup of almonds = 600 milligrams
- 1 cup of soybeans = 460 milligrams
- 8-ounce glass of calcium-fortified orange juice = 300 milligrams
- 1 cup of SoyDream Beverage Original Enriched = 300 milligrams
- 1 cup of sunflower seeds = 260 milligrams
- 10 dried figs = 269 milligrams
- 3 ounces of salmon = 203 milligrams
- ½ cup of collards = 179 milligrams
- broccoli = 178 milligrams
- cornbread = 133 milligrams

If your children are allergic or sensitive to dairy products, the following is a list of ingredients that indicate the use of dairy in a food: Artificial butter flavour, butter, butterfat, buttermilk, casein, caseinates, curds, custards, half and half, hydrolysates, lactalbumin, lactose, nougat, pudding, rennet casein, sour creams, sour milk solids, whey, yogurt.

If you choose to include a certain amount of dairy products in your children's diet, it is wise to wait until they are approximately two years old before introducing them. A later introduction will ward off the development of future allergies or asthmatic reactions. If possible, purchase organic cow's or goat's milk, yogurt, and cheese free of medications and hormones. Check out this great recipe—it is sure to be a hit with your kids!

Protein Shake for Kids

**YIELDS 1-2 SHAKES
(DEPENDING ON SIZE AND APPETITE OF CHILD)**

1 banana
1 cup soy milk or rice milk
1 cup orange juice
5–10 strawberries, sliced
4 tsp natural peanut butter
1 serving greens+ kids (optional)

Blend on high for 30 seconds in blender. This delicious, creamy, and sweet shake is loaded with protein, minerals, and vitamins that can fill up any child!

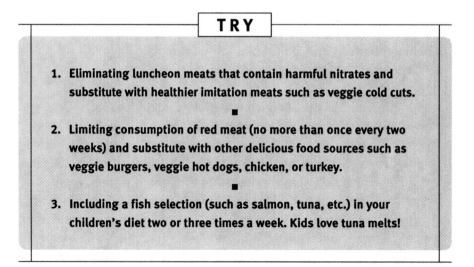

TRY

1. Eliminating luncheon meats that contain harmful nitrates and substitute with healthier imitation meats such as veggie cold cuts.

   ■

2. Limiting consumption of red meat (no more than once every two weeks) and substitute with other delicious food sources such as veggie burgers, veggie hot dogs, chicken, or turkey.

   ■

3. Including a fish selection (such as salmon, tuna, etc.) in your children's diet two or three times a week. Kids love tuna melts!

4. Including nuts as a high-protein snack your kids can munch on. Nuts are slightly higher in fat, so a handful will do! In addition, healthy nut butters (almond, soy, peanut) with jam on whole grain bread are a great lunch.

5. Making yummy omelets or other egg selections as an excellent source of protein for your children. When selecting eggs, choose omega-3 eggs (labeled as such and available in grocery stores).

NOTES

1 National Hot Dog and Sausage Council, www.hot-dog.org

2 Kids Eat Great: Nitrates, www.kidseatgreat.com

3 Hot Dog Cancer Risks and Vitamins, www.ralphmoss.com

4 *TIME* Magazine, Canadian edition, "Playing Chicken with Our Antibiotics," (January 21, 2002).

5 B. Wilcox, C. Wilcox, and M. Suzuki, *The Okinawa Program* (New York: Clarkson Potter Publishers, 2001).

6 Nutrition Action Healthletter 27(10) (December 2000).

7 M. Klaper, *Pregnancy, Children and the Vegan Diet* (Umatilla, FL: Gentle World, Inc., 1987).

8 http://www.milksucks.com/

9 M. Henner, *Total Health Makeover* (New York: ReganBooks, 1998).

10 www.ethicalinvesting.com

11 D. Feskanich, W.C. Willett, M.J. Stampfer, and G.A. Colditz, "Milk, Dietary Calcium, and Bone Fractures in Women: A 12-Year Prospective Study," *American Journal of Public Health* 87 (1997):992–997.

12 R.G. Cumming and R.J. Klineberg, "Case-Control Study of Risk Factors for Hip Fractures in the Elderly," *American Journal of Epidemiology* 139 (1994):493.

CHAPTER 6

Fats: The Good, the Bad, and the Ugly!

F ATS ARE THE third and most misunderstood category of all the macro-nutrients. With an estimated 97 million Americans (55 percent of the population) suffering from obesity (and with Canada's numbers following closely behind), many have come to associate the word fat with heaviness, overindulgence, and unhealthy eating habits. Unfortunately, misleading information and confusing labels have made interpreting the fat game a little tricky. In recent years, consumers have made a definite shift toward "low-fat" products in an attempt to dodge the extra pounds. In reality, these products have had the opposite effect on people's waistlines and actually promote further weight gain. Not only are low-fat foods nutritionally void, they are also filled with an enormous amount of refined flours and sugars to compensate for the lack of taste normally provided by fat. As you now know, refined flours and sugars ring the insulin bell in the body and create chaos with fluctuations in blood sugar levels. This effect results in oversecretion of insulin, excess fat storage, cravings, and mood swings. Void of vitamins and minerals, loaded with sugars, and filled with preservatives, these low-fat products are hindering, not helping, the healthy development of a child. With the increasing numbers of obese adults and children, it is obvious that low-fat foods are clearly not the answer.

Children do not need low-fat products; they need good fat whole foods. Proper neurological development of children is intimately linked with the amount of proper fat intake in their diet. In fact, the human brain is structurally comprised of more than 60 percent fat! Fat is essential for the absorption of vitamins A, D, E, and K and for proper growth and energy production. Just as we need complex carbohydrates and proteins, we also need to consume a certain amount of fat daily. In children, fats should comprise approximately 25–30 percent of their total daily caloric intake. Unlike proteins and carbohydrates, which yield 4 calories per gram, 1 gram of fat yields 9 calories. Hence, as we age and caloric intake needs decline, so do our fat intake requirements. Adults, who require less fat than children, need approximately 20 percent of their total daily caloric intake from fat.

A Closer Look at Fats

To clear up fat's bad rap, it is important to realize that not all fats are created equal. On the positive side, there are fats called essential fatty acids, which are required daily to maintain the health and vitality of every cell in the body. At the other end of the spectrum, there are dangerous fats called trans-fatty acids (tfas), which cause health problems such as clogged arteries, inflammation, neurological disturbances, and an increased risk of heart attacks. The key to understanding fats is to be able to distinguish the good from the bad in your local grocery store. For the purpose of this chapter, fats will be divided into four categories: (1) monounsaturated fats, (2) polyunsaturated fats, (3) saturated fats, and (4) trans-fatty acids.

Monounsaturated fats

Fats are classified according to the number of hydrogen atoms in their molecular structure. Monounsaturated fats are termed as such because they have room to accept one (mono) hydrogen atom. Monounsaturated fats include olive, canola, and peanut oil. In recent years, these oils have shifted into the nutritional limelight, with research showing their use offers significant health benefits. Studies show that individuals who consume the greatest amounts of olive oil, such as those from Mediterranean countries, also tend to have lower incidences of cardiac disease. Monounsaturated fats lower the bad cholesterol (called low-density lipoprotein, or LDL) and have minimal to no effect on the good cholesterol (called high-density lipoprotein, or HDL). There are no specific required daily allowances (RDAS) for fat intake for children; however, most of a child's fat selections should be derived from the monounsaturated group.

When shopping for monounsaturated fat, think olive oil. Extra virgin olive oil is one of the most stable oils for cooking and sautéing and can be easily burned at low heats. This flavorful oil can also be used when preparing salad dressings or mixed with your favorite spices to make a healthy dip for wholesome, grainy bread. When purchasing olive oil, try to choose unrefined, expeller-pressed, extra-virgin (from the first pressing of the olive) olive oil.

Canola oil, first developed in Canada, is also monounsaturated oil derived from genetically modified rapeseed, a member of the mustard family of plants. I do not recommend using this oil in excess. Rapeseed oils are typically used for industrial purposes such as soaps, lubricants, or fuel. Although marketed as healthy, it is questionable as to whether this oil is suitable for human consumption. In rat studies, animals fed canola oil developed fatty degeneration of their hearts, kidneys, adrenals, and thyroid glands. When the canola oil was removed from the rats' diet, the fatty deposits dissolved, but scar tissue remained. Other studies have linked the consumption of canola oil to cases of blindness, emphysema, constipation, cancer, and respiratory distress.[1] Oil from the rapeseed is 100 times more toxic than soy oil. In fact, this oil can be so toxic that it is useful as an insect repellent on crops! Canola oil is the cheapest oil to purchase and is in most processed foods. Until more information is known about this oil's potential side effects, it is best to use olive oil. For baking recipes and sautéing vegetables, fish, chicken, or tofu, olive oil is your best choice.

As a general rule, all oils should be stored in dark, cool places. Monounsaturated oils are typically liquid at room temperature, but solidify when refrigerated.

Avocados – The good fat fruit. Avocados are a unique creamy fruit comprised mostly of monounsaturated fat, and are a tasty and nutrient-packed addition to any child's diet. These fruits were once condemned for containing the bad fat; however, we now know the virtuous disease-fighting attributes of the beloved avocado. If you are unfamiliar with how to find and use avocados, follow these directions:

Avocados can be found in the produce section of most grocery stores. Hold an avocado and gently squeeze it. If the flesh feels soft, it is ripe and perfect for slicing. If you make a dent in the skin of the avocado, it is likely too ripe for slicing, but is perfect for mashing up into a delicious guacamole dip.

After purchasing avocados, it is best to store them at room temperature until they soften. Cut the fruit lengthwise, separate the halves, and remove the pit. If you are mashing up an avocado for a dip, score the green flesh of the fruit with a fork while it is still in the skin. Sprinkle it with lemon juice or keep the pit in the dip or avocado half to prevent browning. Here are some ways to use avocado in your child's diet:

- Add slices of avocado to a veggie or tuna sandwich, wrap, or pita.

- Add avocado chunks to a salad.

- Serve healthy nacho chips and delicious guacamole dip.

- Cut avocados in half, sprinkle with sea salt, and let your children eat it with a spoon.

- Add avocado pieces to omelets with salsa for taste.

Guacamole

SERVES 3–4

4 avocados
5–8 tbsp salsa (mild, medium, or hot, depending on preference)
¼–½ tsp cumin (spice)
½ tsp crushed garlic
½ tsp lemon juice

Mash up green flesh of avocado with fork until creamy. Add salsa, cumin, and garlic, and mix. Add a small amount of lemon juice to prevent browning. Enjoy!

Polyunsaturated Fats

Polyunsaturated fats have room to accept more than one hydrogen atom, hence the term poly. These fats are liquid at room temperature and are found in vegetable oils such as sunflower, sesame, soybean, corn, and safflower oil. It was once thought that these oils were a much healthier alternative to saturated fats because they were derived from a vegetable source. Current research shows that this is not true. Although polyunsaturated oils appear to lower the levels of LDL, the bad cholesterol, they also lower the levels of HDL, the good cholesterol. These types of oils are not healthful and should only be present in minimal amounts in a child's diet.

Among the polyunsaturated fats, there are two exceptions—omega-3 and omega-6 essential fatty acids (EFAs)—that are extremely beneficial to health. EFAs cannot be produced by the body and must be obtained through diet.

- Omega-3 EFA, also called alpha-linolenic acid, is broken down into easily absorbable units called eicosapentaenoic acid (EPA) and docosahexaenoic acid (DHA). Rich sources of omega-3 fatty acid are, fish oil, flaxseed oil, hemp oil, walnuts, cold-water fish (salmon, tuna, mackerel, herring, sardines), sesame seeds, omega-3 eggs, and a variety of other nuts and seeds.

- Omega-6, also called linoleic acid, is broken down into easily absorbable units called GLA (gamma-linoleic acid) and DGLA (dihomogamma linoleic acid). Examples of omega-6 oils are primrose oil and borage oil.

Of their many roles in the body, omega-3 and omega-6 convert into hormone-like compounds called prostaglandin. The breakdown of prostaglandins can take three various pathways called PGE1, PGE2, and PGE3. All three prostaglandin pathways have essential roles, and when they function properly, they enable the body to maintain its homeostatic balance. A problem arises when the PGE2 pathway is overtriggered from eating the wrong foods. In a nutshell, PGE1 and PGE3 are the "good" inflammatory pathways that protect the body from invaders with immune-building properties. PGE2 is the "bad" inflammatory pathway that can lead to too much inflammation and the development of certain disorders such as allergies, asthma, and arthritis. How does PGE2 get overtriggered? By eating too many omega-6 foods. The North American diet is extremely high in omega-6 vegetable oils found in processed goodies, making it very difficult for the body to utilize the small amount of omega-3 we do get from food. There is a delicate balance between omega-6 and omega-3, with the ideal balance being approximately 4:1 respectively. With increased consumption of omega-6 fatty acids in the last 100 years in the form of vegetable oils such as safflower, sunflower, corn, and soybean oil, this ratio has shifted dramatically. Today, in most Western diets, the average ratio of omega 6:omega-3 ranges from 20:1 to 30:1. When the scales are tipped due to the ingestion of saturated fats, trans-fatty acids, or too much omega-6 in the diet, an excess of the "bad" PGE2 prostaglandins are produced. In summary, too much omega-6 in the diet can result in a deficiency of omega-3 and an overproduction of the PGE2 pathway, which can cause asthma, allergies, and arthritis. Thus, the goal is to increase your child's intake of omega-3 essential fatty acids to maintain a proper balance.

In the pediatric populations, omega-3 EFA deficiencies are very common, yet they go largely undiagnosed. Numerous studies have linked a deficiency of essential fatty acids with attention deficit disorder, allergies, and poor motor skills. Consider the following research findings:

- In one study, subjects with lower compositions of total omega-3 fatty acids had significantly more behavior problems, temper tantrums, learning, health, and sleep problems than did those with high proportions of omega-3 fatty acids.[2]

- Another study found that fifty-three subjects with attention deficit hyperactivity disorder had significantly lower concentrations of key fatty acids in the plasma polar lipids and in blood cell total lipids than did the forty-three control subjects.[3]

- Experimental evidence in animals has shown that the effect of essential fatty acid deficiency during early brain development is damaging and permanent.[4]

News reports encourage the public to increase their salmon, tuna, or mackerel intake to raise their levels of omega-3s which are critical for proper nervous system development, for cell membrane integrity, and for proper brain function. Every living cell in the body requires essential fatty acids to rebuild and produce new cells. Essential fatty acids and their derivatives also play a critical role in the proper functioning of the immune system, energy levels, and regulate appropriate anti-inflammatory responses.

The most common signs and symptoms of omega-3 EFA deficiencies in children are:

- Allergies
- Attention deficit disorder (ADD) or attention deficit hyperactivity disorder (ADHD)
- Dandruff
- Dry eyes
- Dry skin

- Eczema
- Hyperactivity
- Irritability
- Fatigue
- Frequent infections
- Learning disabilities
- Poor immune system function
- Poor wound healing

Although they are incredibly nutritious, EFAs are extremely sensitive and cannot exist in processed foods without going rancid quickly. Thus, these foods do not have a long shelf life and must be eaten directly from their source in live, fresh foods. It is often difficult for busy parents and kids to have daily access to omega-3 rich foods. Therefore, I recommend supplementing a child's diet with a high-quality flaxseed oil or fish oil on a daily basis. Both oils are incredibly rich sources of omega-3 fatty acids. One teaspoon per day of flaxseed or fish oil put into your children's juice or shake, or used as a salad dressing or as popcorn topping is all that it takes to fill their requirements. Some children with poor digestive health are unable to break down the omega-3 content from flaxseed oil into its absorbable derivative, DHA, and therefore cannot reap the benefits. Taking fish oil instead of flaxseed oil solves this problem; however, children often dislike the taste of fish oil. If this is the case and your children are old enough, purchase omega-3 fish capsules that have a high percentage of DHA content. Some health food stores even carry omega-3 fish oils that are flavored (such as butterscotch) to disguise any unpleasant taste or odor. (refer to Appendix IV on Dr. Joey's top supplement recommendations for more information.) In addition, ground flaxseeds (they must be ground up to be absorbed) can be sprinkled on top of your child's cereal or salad for an additional essential fatty acid boast. Symptoms related to a deficiency in omega-3 usually respond quickly to supplementation. According to Dr. Leo Galland, author of *Superimmunity for Kids*: "Even when an infant inherits a predisposition for allergies, special protective elements in breast milk, together with EFAS, can delay the onset of allergic illness and greatly reduce its severity."[5]

Breast-feeding mothers can supplement their infants with EFAS by supplementing their own diet with fish oil, flaxseed oil, cold water fish, avocados, nuts, and seeds. Nutrients needed to properly absorb EFAS are: selenium, zinc, carotenes, magnesium, vitamin C, vitamin B3, and vitamin B6. These vitamins and minerals can be obtained by taking a high-quality multivitamin and by eating a diet rich in vegetables, fruits, whole grains, soy, and fish.

Flaxseed oils and fish oils are extremely sensitive to light, air, and oxygen and must be stored in a special way. These oils do best when kept in airtight, dark bottles. If the oil begins to smell, it should be discarded immediately. Healthy oils do not smell, while rancid oils do. Due to their sensitivity to light and temperature, these oils can never be heated. Heating essential fatty acid oils destroys the value of the EFA and produces toxic chemical components that lead to arteriosclerosis and cancer. Remember, the only oil that should be used for frying and sautéing is extra-virgin olive oil.

Saturated Fats

Saturated fats are termed as such because they are completely full or "saturated" with hydrogen atoms. Of all the fats, saturated fats are considered the "bad fats" and should be kept to a minimum in a child's diet. This type of fat is found in animal products, dairy items (cream, whole milk), and tropical oils such as palm and coconut oil. Children's favorite saturated fat picks include ice cream, milk, cheese, hamburgers, hot dogs, pizza, and butter.

The liver uses saturated fat to produce cholesterol. Excessive consumption of saturated fats can raise the level of the bad cholesterol, low-density lipoprotein. Although cholesterol plays a vital role in our bodies, such as maintaining the proper structure of our cell walls and producing the sex hormones estrogen and testosterone, too much cholesterol can have lethal effects on our blood flow. Eating large amounts of saturated fat increases LDL in the body and stiffens and narrows the arterial wall. Only 5 percent of the 25-30 percent total daily fat consumption should be derived from saturated fat. For example, if the average child is consuming 1,800 calories per day, only 3 grams should be derived from saturated fat. The calculation is like this:

1,800 per day multiplied by 0.30 (30 percent from fat)
= 540 calories per day from fat

540 divided by 9 (fat has 9 calories per gram)
= 60 grams

60 multiplied by 0.05
(only 5 percent should be derived from saturated fat)
= 3 grams of fat

For optimal health, it is best to make saturated fats such as ice cream and buttery cookies an occasional treat for your children.

When discussing the issue of saturated fats, the margarine/butter debate must be addressed. In the past, margarine has been heavily marketed as the healthier choice over butter. As you will read in the next section, unless margarine is labeled trans-free, I recommend eliminating this spread from your child's diet. Although manufacturers claim that it is "good for your heart," margarine is a dangerous trans-fatty acid that can lead to plaque buildup in your child's arteries. Although butter is a saturated fat, I believe it is better than margarine. At best, butter is more natural, containing some vital minerals, fat-soluble vitamins, and antifungal and antibacterial properties. When baking with butter, try to use it sparingly in your recipes. Substituting with olive oil or applesauce are other options. Ghee, a clarified butter found in health food stores, is a healthier alternative and is suitable for frying or cooking. In addition, try incorporating healthier spreads such as hummus (chickpea spread), dairy-free or light cream cheese and healthy nut butters into your child's diet. When purchasing nut butters, be aware that most commercial peanut butters are loaded with funny fats and sugar. It is best to avoid using these as staples in your child's lunch. As an alternative, most health food stores carry delicious, naturally sweetened hazelnut, walnut, peanut, and almond butters that make tasty nut butter and jam sandwiches.

Trans-fatty Acids: Buyer Beware!

If saturated fats are considered the bad fats, trans-fatty acids (TFA's) are the "really, really bad fats." TFAs are artificial fats that occur when food technologists alter the chemical structure of a polyunsaturated fat (a vegetable oil) from a round shape to a straight chain. This process is called *hydrogenation* and involves flooding a polyunsaturated fat with an abundant amount of hydrogen atoms at a high temperature. What's the big deal about changing the shape of a little fat molecule? Well, unfortunately, lots. These synthetic fats are known to promote the buildup of plaque in arteries, increase cholesterol levels, promote cancer by causing dangerous defects in cell membranes, and increase the risk of cardiovascular disease. In addition, due to their new shape, trans-fatty acids are extremely difficult for the body to get rid of. Unfortunately, when you start to read labels, you won't find the words trans-fatty acids. To date, the Food and Drug Administration does not require manufacturers to list trans-fatty acids on the label. When it comes to listing ingredients, manufacturers are only required to list the total amount of fat and the saturated fat content. Some products also list the amount of mono- and polyunsaturated fat. So how can you tell if a product contains dangerous trans-fatty acids? If you see the words hydrogenated or "partially hydrogenated oils or fat," move on. It is the equivalent of a trans-fatty acid. Hydrogenated oils or partially hydrogenated oils are found in most packaged, processed products in the grocery store. Margarine, cookies, salad dressing, crackers, pastas, breads, frozen pizzas, and vegetable shortening?—you name it! Seems a little overwhelming doesn't it? Well, it doesn't have to be. Once you get into the habit of identifying and eliminating these products from your child's diet, it will become second nature. You can also sleep a little better, knowing that you are armed with the nutritional information necessary to take control over the quality of your entire family's food choices.

> *Four or five grams of trans-fats a day over a period of fourteen years will increase your heart disease risk by 100 percent.*[6]

Many people have asked me, "If this process is so bad for us, why is it allowed in our grocery stores?" The answer is one word—profit. To the manufacturers of these products, hydrogenation is a very lucrative process. It prolongs shelf life, is cheap to make, and can even turn liquid vegetable oils into artificial spreads such as margarines.

Protect your child's arteries, cell membranes, and heart by becoming fat smart. The next time you purchase foods and snacks from the grocery store, don't let the funny fats make their way into your shopping cart.

CHOLESTEROL

Until recently, it was thought that the intake of high-cholesterol foods such as eggs, shrimp, and meat was responsible for the cholesterol problem experienced by so many adults in North America today. Cholesterol was blamed for conditions such as high blood pressure and the current increase in heart disease and heart attacks. As it turns out, dietary cholesterol isn't really the problem. In fact, only a small percentage of circulating cholesterol in the body (approximately 20 percent) is derived from dietary factors. According to Dr. David Rowland, author of *The Nutritional Bypass*, "80% of people who have had heart attacks did *not* have elevated levels of cholesterol prior to their attack."[7]

Cholesterol is produced by the liver and plays a key role in the maintenance of health. It is involved in the production of hormones, in the conduction of nerve impulses, in the manufacturing of vitamin D, and is necessary for the production of bile. If the diet did not provide cholesterol, the liver would still be able to provide sufficient amounts of cholesterol for survival. The greatest contributors to high blood cholesterol are refined flours and sugars, saturated fats, and trans-fatty acids. Research shows that these sugars and fats cause free radical damage. Free radicals are highly unstable molecules that can create microtears and damage to the walls of arteries. Cholesterol, calcium, and other fillers are laid down to fill the holes created by the free radical damage. It is the process of filling the hole that creates plaque buildup in arterial wall linings, thereby leading to high blood pressure and heart disease. In other words, minimizing the amount of refined sugar, flour, saturated fat, and trans-fatty acids in your child's diet is the best defense against high cholesterol and heart disease. It is not necessary to completely toss out eggs, shrimp, and meat products to keep a child's cholesterol in check. Eating a modest amount of healthy meat and omega-3 eggs (no more than six per week) are excellent sources of protein that only contribute to healthy growth and development. Exercise is also one of the best methods to keep cholesterol at a healthy level.

TRY

1. Including avocados into your children's diet to give them some healthy monounsaturated fats. Make up a yummy guacamole dip with vegetables as a snack or appetizer in any meal.

   ■

2. Using omega-3 eggs for omelets, sandwiches, and french toast.

   ■

3. Avoiding deep-fried foods such as french fries and onion rings. Substitute with some tasty, baked yam french fries loaded with beta-carotene and other vital nutrients!

   ■

4. Including nuts and seeds as snacks for their omega-3 values. Walnuts, pumpkin, sesame, and sunflower seeds are all excellent choices.

   ■

5. If you see the words "hydrogenated" or "partially hydrogenated" on the ingredient list, put down the product! It is filled with chemically harmful fats that will only hinder health.

NOTES

1 www.karinya.com

2 J. Burges, L. Stevens, W. Zhang, and L. Peck. "Long Chain-Polyunsaturated Fatty Acids in Children with Attention-Deficit Hyperactivity Disorder," *The American Journal of Clinical Nutrition* 71(1) (January 2000, 327–330.

3 L. Stevens et al., "Essential Fatty Acid Metabolism in Boys with Attention Deficit Hyperactivity Disorder," *The American Journal of Clinical Nutrition* 62 (1995): 761–768.

4 M. Crawford, "The Role of Essential Fatty Acids in Neural Development: Implications for Perinatal Nutrition," *The American Journal of Clinical Nutrition* 57 (1993): 703S–709S.

5 L. Galland, *Superimmunity for Kids* (New York: Dutton, 1988).

6 *The Globe and Mail*, "Living in the Fast-Food Lane" (July 9, 2002).

7 D. Roland, *The Nutritional Bypass* (Parry Sound: Rowland Publications, 1999).

CHAPTER 7

Sugar and Other Monsters

O N A RECENT VISIT to a local grade school, I was troubled to discover soft drink dispensers in the school cafeteria. When I asked why this non-food was allowed and freely available for kids to purchase, I was told that most schools have them. Upon further researching this issue, I found out that soft drink companies spend millions of dollars annually to place their products and ads in school lunchrooms and auditoriums. The average can of pop, which contains between 6–10 teaspoons of sugar, is readily available for kids to drink! This is totally absurd. We know that sugar suppresses the immune system, creates lack of focus, mood fluctuations, and fatigue. Not really the ideal state for our kids to be in at school, is it? The fact is, white sugar foods have flooded the food industry. According to a CNN report, the consumption of candy in the United States has increased by 50 percent between 1980 and 1995. In addition, soft drink consumption has doubled in the past twenty-five years. *These statistics mean that the average child consumes 29 teaspoons of added refined sugar per day.*[1] With obesity, allergies, and autoimmune conditions on the rise, it is definitely time for parents to take notice and discover the truth about what their children are eating.

SUGAR: THE ANTI-NUTRIENT

Along with refined flours, refined sugar consumption is wreaking havoc on our children's health. Today's child has become addicted to sugary foods and snacks. Similar to addictions to drugs, alcohol, or caffeine, eliminating sugar from children's diets can result in withdrawal symptoms such as intense cravings, tantrums, and mood swings. Providing a child with healthy, natural sweet snacks such as melon cubes, apple slices, or healthy homemade baked goods with natural sweeteners makes this process easier. Adding vegetables, whole grains, and proteins will also help.

It's important to pay attention to your child's cravings. Most people think their cravings for salty or sweet food are normal. Cravings are not normal—they are an indication that your system is out of whack nutritionally and/or biochemically. Luckily, withdrawal symptoms from sugar usually do not last long and other sweet-tasting natural foods can be added back into the diet as a healthier alternative. Withdrawal symptoms normally subside within one to two weeks.

The sugar industry generates over $1 billion per year.

When I first discuss the ills of white sugar consumption with parents, I commonly hear the following remarks:

- "My children do not eat candy."
- "We never add sugar to our food."
- "Our kids do not drink pop."
- "We don't have any white sugar in our house."

Unfortunately, white sugar is in many products unbeknownst to the consumer. Sugar is in cookies, cereals, cola, juices, jams, ketchup, tomato sauce, peanut butter, and even some toothpaste products! It is very difficult for parents to compete with slick advertising campaigns that lure their children toward the latest sugary delight. Of course, companies selling these products know their target audience well—our kids! An increase in sugar consumption means greater profit and success. Food manufacturers know that if they get the kids to want the products, they will likely get the parents to buy them.

It is estimated that refined sugar production is approximately 200 billion pounds per year, and personal consumption, in well-to-do countries, often exceeds 100 pounds per year.[2]

In this chapter, when reviewing the harmful effects of sugar, I will be referring to refined sugars, not naturally occurring sugars such as those in fruit. Although sugar is derived from a natural source, the sugar beet or the sugar cane, it is the process of producing refined sugars that strips away 90 percent of their fibrous material. Similar to refining grains, removing this material also removes the precious vitamins, minerals, and fiber found in the original plant. Sugar derived from the sugar cane or beets is processed into sucrose (table sugar) and appears on our tables as refined, white crystals. With the fiber removed, sugar crystals enter the bloodstream far too quickly, resulting in a heightened insulin response. As you now know, high levels of insulin and the fluctuations of a child's blood sugar can lead to symptoms such as mood swings, weight gain, headaches, and low energy. Chapter 9 focuses on attention deficit disorder and outlines the connection between sugar and mood and discusses how food elimination diets can be beneficial for children suffering from behavioral disorders.

Garbage In, Garbage Out!

A child's immune system is important for the maintenance of health and prevention of illness. There are literally millions of potentially harmful viruses, bacteria, and yeast that our immune systems respond to daily. At school, in the playground, and at birthday parties, a child's immune system is constantly being challenged. This response is normal and advantageous to a child. In fact, these bugs actually strengthen the immune system for similar, future challenges. The cells that fight off infections are called white blood cells. White blood cells are the frontline ammunition used by the immune system to kill off any nasty critters. There are many forms of white blood cells such as lymphocytes, macrophages, B cells, and T cells, that go to work when they first detect an invader. Once the invader is detected, white blood cells will attach themselves to the invader and chomp it up. In addition, the immune system, in its innate wisdom, also creates memory cells that will learn, identify, and then remember specific invaders as a safeguard against future attacks. The next-time your child's systems detect a familiar invader, they will respond more quickly and more efficiently than they did on first detection.

The immune system can be compared to the smooth running of a car's engine. Disturbing one part of the engine such as the carburetor, oil filter, or spark plug can upset the entire functioning of the car. Similar to a car's engine, if the immune system is disturbed, it can upset the surrounding systems, causing a crash in a child's health. This is where sugar comes in. Sugar is one of the major substances that can throw off the immune system, allowing the perfect environment for illness or infection to develop by lowering white blood cell response. In his book, *The Encyclopedia of Natural Medicine*, Michael Murray states: "It is clear, particularly during an infection, that the consumption of simple sugars, even in the form of fruit juice, is deleterious to the host's immune system."[3]

A scale called the leukocytic index is often used to measure how many invaders a white blood cell can kill within an hour. The average leukocytic index number is approximately 13.9. According to Dr. Stoll, author of *Saving Yourself from the Disease-Care Crisis*, within fifteen minutes of consuming approximately 100 grams of refined sugar (the average consumed in an evening meal), the leukocytic index drops to 1.4—meaning the average person loses over 90 percent of immune function! This is important to remember before giving your child suffering from a sore throat a sugary banana Popsicle to suck on. By doing so, you only further reduce his or her much-needed immune response. Instead of white sugary sweets, support your children's systems by providing them with natural immune-enhancing substances such as fruit or natural fruit juice packed with immune-boosting vitamin C.

Soft drinks, containing 40 grams of sugar per 12 ounces, are by far the biggest source of sugar in the average American's diet.

The United States Department of Health recommends no more than 10 teaspoons of sugar per day. In my opinion, because of sugar's immune-suppressing effects, this amount is still far too high. Consider the sugar value found in some of kids' favorite food items:

Sugar Values in Some Foods

Food	Teaspoons	% Daily Value
Snickers bar, 2.1 oz	5¾	58
Low-fat, fruit-flavored yogurt, 8 oz	7	70
Pepsi, 12 oz	10¼	103
Pancake syrup, ¼ cup	10¼	103
Hostess Lemon Fruit Pie, 4½ oz	11½	115
McDonald's Vanilla Shake, 20 oz	12	120
Cinnabon, 7¼ oz	12¼	123
Strawberry Passion Awareness Fruitopia, 20 oz	17¾	178
Dairy Queen Mr. Misty Slush, 32 oz	28	280

Sources: Manufacturers, USDA, CSPI analyses and/or estimates.[4]
Center for Science in the Public Interest, August 1999

Acid versus Alkaline

Another problem caused by sugar intake is the overly acidic environment it creates in the body. Illness and disease proliferate in an acidic, not alkaline (the opposite of acidic), environment. The scale used to measure the acid/alkaline balance is called the pH (potential of hydrogen) scale. The normal pH of the body is approximately 7.0. Anything higher shifts you to a more alkaline state and anything lower shifts you to a more acidic state. You can test your family's pH levels by purchasing pH paper from your local health food store. Don't eat for one hour prior to the test. Simply rinse your mouth with water and wait five minutes. Place a piece of pH paper in your mouth and moisten it with saliva. A color scale will be included with your pH paper to indicate your results. Yellow typically means acidic and green/blue is closer to alkaline (a normal pH).

When the body is overly acidic, it attempts to maintain balance by using a basic buffer to counteract the acidity. For example, calcium (the most abundant basic mineral in the body) can be leached from the bones in an attempt to maintain a normal pH. This is another example of how sugar creates a nutrient debt. If I haven't already convinced you of the ills of refined sugar, here is a condensed list of more health problems that sugar can cause:

- Acne
- Candidiasis (yeast infections)
- Cholesterol increase
- Contributes to Type II diabetes
- Depression
- Desensitization to insulin response
- Diarrhea and/or constipation
- Eczema
- Food allergies and intolerances
- Hyperactivity
- Hypo- or hyperglycemia (low and high blood sugar respectively)
- Immune system suppression
- Low energy
- Mood swings
- Obesity and weight gain

- Severe PMS symptoms
- Stomach upset
- Tooth decay

How to Avoid Sugar

Labels list ingredients in descending order by weight. If a product's first ingredient is sugar, the percentage of sugar in that product is greater than any other, leaving little room for proper nutrition. When reading labels, pay attention to the following words, which indicate the presence of a refined sugar: glucose, sucrose, fructose, high fructose corn syrup, white sugar, brown sugar, granulated sugar, powdered sugar, icing sugar, and dextrose.

There is some debate about the health benefits of refined fructose (not the naturally occurring fructose in fruit). Fructose is often recommended for diabetics because of its low glycemic index rating (GI = 20). This sugar enters the bloodstream very slowly and does not cause a heightened insulin response. Fructose has also been shown to increase insulin sensitivity by 34 percent, which is good news for diabetics who have become insulin insensitive. On the negative side, there are reports that an over consumption of fructose can increase LDL, the bad cholesterol, so I recommend using fructose in moderation along with the other natural sugars.

As for brown sugar, there is a widespread misconception that it is healthier than white sugar. Most brown sugars are merely white sugars that have been cleverly disguised. Brown sugar is just as refined as white sugar with a bit of molasses, sugar syrup, and caramel coloring added to darken it. Tricky isn't it?

Healthier Options

Children definitely lead the pack in terms of being sugar monsters. However, kids are not born with a natural sweet tooth. Sweet tooth syndrome and cravings are the result of the chemical imbalances caused by eating a large amount of refined foods. To a child, sugar represents fun and excitement such as Halloween, birthday cakes, and holidays. Providing your children a healthier diet does not necessarily mean eliminating all their sweet-tasting goodies. There is still a way for them to enjoy sweet, whole foods without experiencing the harmful effects that white sugar creates. You will be thrilled to discover that there are many healthier alternatives to white sugar that taste equally or even more delicious. The first step to switching your children to a naturally sweet diet is to clean out your cupboards. This will be a very enlightening exercise to perform. Now that you are an informed label reader, you will be shocked to find out how many products contain white sugar. By removing the junk from your home, your children will not feel as tempted or deprived. Children quickly become accustomed to the idea of eating healthily at at home and having occasional treats outside the home. How strictly you enforce a white sugar-free diet is entirely up to you. This is where the 80-20 rule is very useful. Exceptions to this rule are if your children suffer from allergies, asthma, or other illnesses. In these cases, it is best to go cold turkey in eliminating sugar until the condition clears. Use natural sweets to help them get over the withdrawal symptoms and make them healthier homemade snacks so they do not feel deprived. Trust yourself, you know your children the best.

> *When looking for brown sugar, the word unrefined is very important. Certain brown sugars are merely white sugar plus coloring.*

So, what are healthier sweet options for your children? Fresh fruit is always one of the best selections for the entire family. They are naturally sweet and filled with vitamins and minerals. The key to having your kids eat more fruit is to make it readily available for them to grab as snacks. Try cutting up some apples, keeping clementines on the kitchen table, or making frozen Popsicles from natural fruit juices. If they become familiar and accustomed to fruit as a viable snack food, they will soon learn to eat it. Here are other natural sweeteners that provide more minerals and vitamins than white sugar:

- Pure maple syrup (once opened, it must be stored in the fridge)
- Molasses (the dark syrup that's left over after sugar has been refined; it's very concentrated, so only a little is needed for baking)
- Barley malt
- Rice syrup
- Dates

- Demerara –(a traditional unrefined sugar, produced to have larger and crunchier crystals than granulated sugar)
- Turbinado brown sugar (light brown, granulated sugar)
- Sucanat (granulated cane juice)

Barley malt's taste is very sweet and mild, while rice syrup is a little lighter and thinner. All of these substitutes can be used in baking recipes instead of sugar.

Another healthier option is the non-caloric herb stevia. This herb, native to Paraguay, has been used for centuries. Stevia is about 100 to 400 times sweeter than sugar. It is heat stable and appropriate for cooking or baking. Some report a slight licorice aftertaste in baked goods made with stevia. Ironically, this herb has generated great controversy. The FDA has attempted to label stevia as an unsafe food product. Prior to 1980, stevia was on the FDA's Generally Regarded as Safe list. Curiously, stevia was removed from this list at the same time aspartame made its way onto the scene. There have been no ill effects reported due to the usage of stevia.[5] On the other hand, aspartame is a toxic substance that should be strictly eliminated from your children's diets. Cooking with stevia takes practice. If you are interested in becoming more familiar with this herb, *The Stevia Cookbook* by Ray Sahelian, MD, is available at most bookstores.

THE OTHER MONSTERS

Yeast

An excessive amount of sugar and refined carbohydrates creates the perfect environment for harmful yeast, called candida, to overgrow. A certain amount of candida naturally lives in the microflora of the digestive system; however, when an overgrowth occurs, it can be harmful to a child's health. Persistent yeast can burrow into a child's digestive system, creating a multitude of symptoms including:

- Allergic shiners (dark circles under eyes)
- Brain fog
- Depression
- Dry eyes

- Extreme fatigue
- Frequent infections
- Headaches
- Irritability/mood swings
- Sluggish digestion
- Skin rashes/eczema/hives
- Sugar cravings
- Unexplained weight gain
- White-coated tongue or thrush
- Yeast infections

Clearing your children of yeast takes time, effort, and education. A yeast-free diet is very restrictive and can be quite hard for both parents and children to follow. For starters, improving digestion and avoiding all refined foods is the first step to take. It is also best to include a supplement of the good bacteria, a probiotic called acidophilus or bifidus when trying to clear children of yeast. Children under the age of two require bifidus, while children over the age of two do better with an acidophilus supplement. These supplements are live cultures and must be stored in the fridge. It is best to take these good bacteria on an empty stomach. Most traditional medical doctors do not check for the presence of candida in children's system; however, it is a condition that must be considered. If you suspect your children are suffering from an overgrowth of yeast, consult a health care practitioner with experience in this field such as a naturopath, nutritionist, holistic medical doctor, etc. A qualified health care professional will be able to design a yeast-free diet and supplement program appropriate for your children.

Refined sugars and carbohydrates are not the only causes of an overgrowth of yeast. An increase in the use of broad-spectrum antibiotics in the younger population is the number one factor that kills off the good bacteria and creates the perfect environment for candida to grow.

Additives

It is estimated that the average person consumes approximately 11 pounds of food additives per year in the form of preservatives, colors, waxes, and emulsifiers. Children are even more susceptible to these foreign chemicals because of their smaller bodies and their developing systems. Knowing who will react to these additives and who will not is a guessing game. Further, the long-term health effects of exposure to these toxins is unknown and can only be guessed. The stakes are far too high. Our children are not guinea pigs and their future health should not be gambled with. Although at first eliminating additives and preservatives from your children's diet may seem like an enormous effort, it can be done. Even reducing their toxic load slightly can have huge benefits. Here are the most common food additives that can be found in every grocery store.

Aspartame

Aspartame, otherwise called NutraSweet, Equal, Spoonful, or Equal Measure, is found in over 5,000 food products such as sweeteners, baked goods, chewing gum, diet carbonated beverages, desserts, candy, and even some pharmaceuticals. As aspartame is approximately 200 times sweeter than regular sugar, a much smaller amount of it is used to sweeten foods. This food additive, discovered by accident in 1965 by chemist James Schlatter, was originally meant to be a peptic ulcer drug. In 1981, the Food and Drug Administration, in a rushed decision, approved aspartame as safe for use in foods.

Aspartame consists of three components: the amino acid phenylalanine, aspartic acid, and methanol, otherwise known as wood alcohol. Methanol is toxic in humans, even when consumed in relatively small amounts. Reactions to aspartame toxicity can be immediate (within forty-eight hours) in children or can occur several days or several years later. Some of the most documented side effects of aspartame are: headaches, migraines, dizziness, seizures, nausea, numbness, muscle spasms, heart palpitations, vision problems, and anxiety. According to researchers, the following conditions can be triggered or worsened by consuming aspartame: epilepsy, multiple sclerosis, chronic fatigue syndrome, fibromyalgia, Parkinson's, birth defects, and diabetes.[6] Although some diabetic programs and associations still recommend aspartame as an alternative to sugar, it is not a safe option. This food additive is a toxic chemical that should be

> *Since 1980, consumption of artificial sweeteners and rates of obesity have both soared.*

completely eliminated from the diet. If your children are suffering from a myriad of bizarre symptoms that doctors can't diagnose, check their diet for aspartame.

Caffeine

Sodas are currently the number one item purchased in American grocery stores today, with average sales generating approximately $12 billion dollars annually. We have all seen kids lining up with their Big Gulp cups at the local hangout, waiting for a second or third free refill. Not only are these drinks loaded with sugar, they are also heavily laden with caffeine.

Caffeine is a central nervous system stimulant that is added to soda pops, coffee, tea, and chocolate. As a stimulant, it can cause the following effects in children: sleep disturbances, anxiety, heart palpitations, hyperactivity, calcium loss, and dehydration. As the largest selling drug in the world, caffeine is addictive, so its removal from the diet creates withdrawal symptoms. According to Stephen Cherniske, author of *Caffeine Blues*:

> Health experts are most worried about the effects of soft drink consumption on children. After ingesting soft drinks, they may have high levels of caffeine for many hours. The cumulative effects derived from consuming soft drinks throughout the day are completely unknown, but it may be no coincidence that cases of hyperactivity and ADD have grown to epidemic proportions at the same time soft drinks have become the dominant fluid intake for many children.[7]

Caffeine also has a high level of acidity. As you now know, an overly acidic environment will leach minerals such as calcium from the body. Harvard researchers found that caffeine leaches small amounts of calcium from the bones, possibly increasing the risk of bone fractures.[8] As children's bones are growing and developing, this is a real concern. It is recommended that children consume much less than 100 milligrams of caffeine per day (two cans of the average soda). This level is far exceeded by most children.

One glass of water is lost for every cup of coffee or can of pop consumed. Replace caffeine fluids with clean water and natural fruit juices.

It is best for children to drink at least four to six glasses of fresh water per day.

Herbicides and Pesticides

Pesticides and herbicides were first introduced in the 1950s to kill any potentially harmful bugs that found their way into our food source. The hypothesis was that while these chemicals would kill bugs, they would have no harmful effects on humans. If you really stop to think about it, how can that make sense? If a chemical kills a microorganism, regardless of its size, it surely will have some effect on other species. Chemicals and pesticides are not used sparingly either. It is estimated that thirty times more pesticides are used now as compared to fifty years ago, and there has been a 20 percent increase in overall pests![9] Consider some of the following statistics:

- The Canadian Institute for Children's Health has found that children are increasingly at risk of serious diseases from pesticides. The study also found that pesticides have *not* been evaluated for their potential to affect brain development.[10]

- Cancer rates have increased 25 percent in children since 1975.[11]

- In 1999, the Food and Drug Administration's residue-monitoring program found pesticide residues on 38 percent of domestic grain products, 29 percent of fish/shellfish, 60 percent of fruits, and 29 percent of vegetables.[12]

Truthfully, researchers and medical professionals are not sure of the long-term health and environmental effects of pesticides and herbicides. What we do know for sure is that certain pesticides are carcinogenic substances, meaning they cause cancer. As a preventative measure, purchase certified organic produce or buy your fruits and vegetables from a local organic farmer. Although this is likely more expensive, it is the best way to ensure minimal consumption of unwanted chemicals. If certified organic produce is not an option, thoroughly wash and scrub all of your fruits and vegetables before eating. While this will not remove all the chemicals, it does remove some. Grapefruit seed extract, a powerful astringent that can be used to wash produce, can be purchased at most health food stores.

Food Dyes

In the past, foods were colored for cosmetic purposes with natural plant and vegetables compounds such as beets for the color red and chlorophyll for the color green. After World War II, chemists developed synthetic food dyes from artificial petroleum-based ingredients. Unlike natural sources of color, synthetic coloring was cost effective, reproducible, and had unlimited shelf life. In Canada, there are eight approved food dyes regulated by the Canadian Food Inspection Agency, and in the United States there are seven food dyes regulated by the Food and Drug Administration. The names of the various color dyes in North America include the following:

- FD&C Red #40 (Canada and United States)
- FD&C Blue #1 (Canada and United States)
- FD&C Blue #2 (Canada and United States)
- FD&C Red #3 (Canada and United States)
- FD&C Yellow #5, Tartrazine (Canada and United States)
- FD&C Yellow #6 (Canada and United States)
- FD&C Green #3 (United States)
- Amaranth (red) (Canada)
- Fast Green FCF (Canada)[13]

Food dyes fall into the anti-nutrient category, meaning they have zero nutritional value and may be hazardous to health. These synthetic dyes are usually found in foods that children love to snack on such as licorice, cupcakes, baked goods, sugary breakfast cereals, and are even found in certain vitamins, pharmaceuticals, and toothpastes. Current research on food dye consumption shows mixed results; certain studies show no effect, while others studies demonstrate that food dye consumption can worsen behavioral problems such as attention deficit disorder. Parents report that after their children consume red or yellow dyes, symptoms of irritability, tantrums, belligerence, and antisocial behavior worsen. In 1970, Dr. Feingold, author of *The Feingold Diet*, conducted the largest analysis on food dye consumption. His results showed dramatic improvements in children's behavior (between 32 and 60 percent) after eliminating artificial dyes and additives from their diet. Follow-up studies, although questionable in design, have not been able to reproduce Dr. Feingold's results. Of all the food dyes, tartrazine (also called FD&C Yellow #5) is one of the most problematic in children and may cause the worsening or development of allergies, asthma, hives, and thyroid tumors.

The monitoring, research, and safety of food dyes is not well documented or managed. Children are bombarded with enough toxic chemicals in the air they breathe, the water they drink, and they food they eat. Eliminating petroleum-based dyes is one small step that can reduce your children's toxic load.

Butylated Hydroxytoluene (BHT) and Butylated Hydroxyanisole (BHA)

Butylated hydroxyanisole (BHA) and butylated hydroxytoluene (BHT) are preservatives used to keep the flavor and color in food and to prevent rancidity. Both are found in foods high in fats and oils such as meats, butter, beer, snack food, dehydrated potatoes, and in chewing gum. These two preservatives have been implicated in various health problems such as cancer, tumor growth in laboratory animals, increase in liver enzymes, bronchospasm, and behavioral disorders. BHT and BHA are banned in certain countries such as Japan, and are not permitted in baby food.

Monosodium Glutamate (MSG)

There is a misconception that if you avoid eating Chinese food, you can avoid MSG. This is simply not so. In fact, in recent years, several Chinese restaurants have completely eliminated MSG from their establishments. Unfortunately, MSG is found in a high percentage of processed, bagged, or bottled food. However, just because a label does not list the words monosodium glutamate as part of its ingredients does not necessarily mean that it is free of MSG. Ingredients such as autolyzed yeast and hydrolyzed protein contain a percentage of monosodium glutamate.[14] Not really fair game for parents, is it?

Why should MSG be completely eliminated from every child's diet? MSG is of great concern because it crosses a safety net, called the blood-brain barrier, which separates the brain from the rest of the body. Signs and symptoms associated with MSG consumption are well documented and include: headaches, migraines, stomach aches, irritable bowel disease, panic attacks, heart palpitations, mental confusion, hyperactivity, and neurological disorders that can mimic Parkinson's, Alzheimer's, amyotropic lateral sclerosis, and fibromyalgia. MSG tricks the brain into thinking that the food you are eating tastes good, causing you to consume more and more of the product. Even if your children do not show any symptoms, it is best to minimize your family's exposure to MSG. If you suspect your children are reacting to MSG and would like further information, *Battling the MSG Myth* by Debby Anglesey is an excellent resource.

TRY

1. Eliminating food ingredients that you cannot pronounce! Remember, there is no such thing as "empty calories." Every food eaten can help or hinder your children's health.

   ■

2. Getting your children used to the taste of natural sweetness by always having cut-up fruit available for snacking.

   ■

3. Checking for the amount of sugar listed in food sources. If the first or second words are glucose, sucrose, white sugar, fructose, or high fructose corn syrup, the product is loaded with sugar and can impair your children's immune systems.

   ■

4. Eliminating sugarless gum that has been sweetened with aspartame. Chewing gum is one of the most common ways aspartame is absorbed. Substitute with naturally sweetened candies, lollipops, or gum available at most health food stores.

   ■

5. Keeping pop out of your children's diet. Fresh, clean water or natural juices are your best bet. Refer to Appendix I for healthy juice selections.

NOTES

1 CNN, "Are Kids Eating Too Much Sugar?" (October 22, 1999) www.cnn.com.

2 "Refined Sugar Products and Their Effect on the Body and Mind," www.trufax.org.

3 M. Murray and J. Pizzorno, *Encyclopaedia of Natural Medicine* (New York: Prima Publishing, 1991).

4 www.cspinet.org

5 www.raysahelian.com

6 "Aspartame, Cause of Disease? NutraSweet, Equal, Spoonful, Equal Measure," www.curezone.com.

7 S. Cherniske, *Caffeine Blues: Wake Up to the Hidden Dangers of America's #1 Drug* (New York, Warner, 1998).

8 http://abcnews.go.com

9 B. Jenson and M. Anderson, *Empty Harvest* (New York: Avery Publishing Group, 1990).

10 www.ecochem.com

11 www.ecochem.com

12 www.ecochem.com

13 www.calicofoods.com

14 www.msgmyth.com

PART III

Childhood Illnesses

We are indeed much more than we eat,
but what we eat can help us to become much
more than whom we are.—ADELE DAVIS

IN THE LAST FIFTY to 100 years, childhood illnesses and diseases have taken a dramatic shift. Children used to suffer and die from tuberculosis, pneumonia, and malnutrition, today's pediatric epidemics include obesity, Type II diabetes, asthma, and allergies. This shift is largely due to the changes in the quality and quantity of the food our kids are consuming daily. Diseases are no longer developing because of poor sanitation or a lack of food supplies. On the contrary, most of the illnesses discussed in the following chapters are what I refer to as the gluttony diseases of the twenty-first century.

The following section will identify the major diseases occurring in children throughout North America and the nutritional contributors to their development. This section has been designed to offer easy nutritional steps for providing effective, natural methods to deal.

CHAPTER 8

Childhood Obesity and Type II Diabetes

THE NUMBER OF obese and overweight children in North America has escalated to epidemic proportions. Obesity rates for children between the ages of seven and thirteen have more than doubled from 1981 to 1996.[1] Today, it is currently estimated that one out of every five children in the United States is obese. Researchers and health care professionals are now scrambling for solutions to fix the obesity problem. Unfortunately, there is no magic bullet. There are many factors responsible for the extra pounds our children are carrying today. In fact, only 1 percent of all obesity cases diagnosed are due to a genetic predisposition. The remaining 99 percent are caused by two major contributing factors:

1. the quality and quantity of food children are consuming daily, and
2. a dramatic drop in daily physical activity.

Rather than eating fresh fruits, vegetables, and whole grains, kids' favorite foods are french fries, hot dogs, cheesy pizza, and sugary fruit roll-ups. Instead of playing outside or running in the park, children are mindlessly munching in front of the television or computer screen for hours. Recently, I saw an ad for a sugary, chemical-filled cereal that included a CD-rom as a bonus at the bottom of the cereal box. Not only is this product filled with unhealthy ingredients such as food coloring, sugar, and partially hydrogenated vegetable oils, the bonus gift of a CD-rom will keep your children in front of a computer for hours. The real irony is that the manufacturers of this cereal were marketing the product as a healthy choice for kids because it had been fortified with a little vitamin B3. Sadly, products like these will only further weight gain, diabetes, and heart disease, possibly shaving years off a child's life. Let's take back control over our food and stop this insanity!

When looking at the disease rates in our children, it is evident that the combination of poor food choices and lack of activity are physically and mentally risky. Studies show that obese children and teenagers have a higher risk of suffering from emotional problems such as low self-esteem, depression, anxiety, and obsessive-compulsive disorder.[2] In addition to scarring psychological consequences, we are also now seeing adult-like diseases in our youth. Overweight children are more than twice as likely to develop high blood pressure or heart disease, Type II diabetes, and even some cancers. An immediate change must be made to curb the trend toward a future generation of obese adults. If not dealt with, we run the risk of creating irreversible, costly health problems in our youth.

> *Overweight adolescents have a 70 percent chance of becoming overweight or obese adults. This increases to 80 percent if one or both parents are overweight or obese.*

WHERE HAVE WE GONE WRONG?

While it is true that there is no single dietary culprit responsible for childhood obesity, there are certain foods in our grocery stores that are causing kids (and adults!) to unknowingly pack on extra pounds. The shift from whole to refined and processed foods is definitely one of the biggest contributors to the problem. Stripping a natural grain of its fiber, adding refined sugars, and adding chemicals such as MSG, which stimulate the brain to eat more and more, is a one-way ticket to weight gain for most. Although the effects of refined foods and sugars have been reviewed in the previous chapters, the following is a summary of the top five foods that are causing the epidemic of obesity in kids:

1. **White, refined flour products:** bread, bagels, cereals, muffins, crackers, cakes, cookies, doughnuts, and granola bars

2. **White sugar:** soda, candy, cookies, cakes, gum, and ketchup

3. **Hydrogenated and/or partially hydrogenated fat:** margarine, refined vegetable oils, chips, most microwave popcorn, cookies

4. **Processed fast foods:** luncheon meats, french fries, burgers, micro-wave pizza

5. **Saturated fat:** cheese, hot dogs, hamburgers, luncheon meats

As you now know, white refined flour and sugar will overtrigger the release of the hormone insulin, secreted by the pancreas. When excess insulin is secreted because of faulty food choices, it is stored as fat. With the perpetual intake of highly refined foods, which are the mainstay of an average child's diet, cell receptors become insensitive to the amount of insulin released. In order to compensate for the insulin insensitivity, the body will secrete more and more insulin to deal with the glucose (sugar) from the food. As a general rule, more insulin = more fat storage. In order to conceptualize the amount of insulin secreted by a healthy body versus a body that has become insulin insensitive, consider the following statistic by one of the world's foremost authorities in nutritional and natural medicine, Dr. Michael Murray: "It is estimated that healthy individuals secrete approximately 31 units of insulin daily, while the obese type II diabetic secretes an average of 114 units daily."[3]

The state of insulin insensitivity is the first step toward the development of obesity and Type II diabetes. Luckily, this process can be halted and even reversed in children when proper dietary guidelines are introduced.

TYPE II DIABETES

Type II diabetes, usually referred to as adult-onset diabetes, is now occurring in younger generations. In the United States, 300,000 children were diagnosed in 2001, and the numbers are continuing to rise. In a study published in *The Journal of the American Academy of Pediatrics*, it was found that approximately 85 percent of all Type II cases in children were caused by obesity. In another recent study published in *The New England Journal of Medicine*, researchers tested obese children (those with a body mass index in the ninety-fifth percentile) for evidence of impaired glucose tolerance. Impaired glucose tolerance means that the body is unable to use sugar properly and the sugar levels in the blood spike higher than normal following a meal. This is considered the first step toward the development of Type II diabetes. Of the kids ages four to ten, 25 percent had impaired glucose tolerance. This translates into one out of every four children showing signs of Type II diabetes![4] This finding is alarming and requires immediate action because of the complications that can result from Type II diabetes including:

- **Atherosclerosis:** the buildup of plaque in the arterial walls leading to the development of heart disease and/or stroke.

- **Diabetic neuropathy:** loss of nerve function resulting in muscular pain, weakness, numbness and tingling.

- **Diabetic retinopathy:** a serious eye disease that can result in blindness; diabetic retinopathy is the leading cause of blindness in the United States.

- **Diabetic nephropathy:** kidney diseases.

- **Foot ulcers:** due to loss of nerve function and blood supply.

Although children may not show overt symptoms of Type II diabetes, dangerous changes that are not yet detectable may be occurring. The fact that diabetes is now being detected in children as young as age three should sound an alarm bell in our medical system. I realize that making changes to a child's diet and weight takes time and effort; however, it is the only way to prevent and reverse the development of this disease.

Is My Child Overweight?

Obesity commonly develops between the ages of five and six or during adolescence. How do you know if your children are overweight or obese? Generally, children are not considered obese until their weight is at least 10 percent higher than what is recommended for their average height and weight. When determining the normal body weight for children, doctors often refer to the body mass index (BMI). The BMI is also used to assess healthy body weight in adults. Recently, the Center for Disease Control has created a version of the BMI scale that addresses the pediatric population ranging in the ages from two to twenty. In order to determine if your children are in the normal range of their BMI, visit www.keepkidshealthy.com to calculate their BMIs.

The BMI is just a tool. Other factors should be considered when determining a healthy weight for a child. Many parents use their children's appearance to determine if they are overweight or not. When doing so, please exercise caution. As a society, we are too inclined to equate thinness with health. It is important for parents to examine their own health perceptions and to reject this notion. If your children are slightly heftier than their schoolmates, assure them that kids come in all different shapes and sizes. There is no perfect figure for a child, and if he or she is healthy, size should be celebrated, not judged. Other health checks to consider when determining healthy body weight are the following:

- Can your children run to the bus or climb the stairs without losing their breath?
- Do they complain of low energy levels?
- Do they resist active play?
- Are their blood pressures within normal range?

Your children's physical condition can help you determine if they are at healthy weights or not. If you are still unsure or concerned, consult your doctor for a complete physical.

Should My Child Go on a Diet?

Research clearly demonstrates that 95 percent of all diets fail. Instead of a diet, your goal should be to shift your children to a state of health and wellness. It is also best to explore if their excess weight may be due to an emotional problem. It is not uncommon for children to use food as comfort. Are they fitting in at school? Is something bothering them at home? Are they eating when they are sad or bored? Start by opening up the lines of communication with them to see if there is an underlying cause for their eating patterns.

With the alarming number of children suffering from obesity, it is obvious that there is more involved than just lack of discipline with food. Children should not be blamed for unknowingly eating themselves into an overweight or obese state. It is important to assure an overweight or obese child that their current physical state is reversible when the necessary steps are taken. Instead of focusing on a diet that will ultimately fail and lead to more weight gain, start incorporating techniques that do work.

> *"At age sixteen my son was considerably overweight. He would easily lose his breath while climbing the stairs and when playing with friends. Our entire family simply eliminated white flours and pops and substituted in fresh water, more fruits and vegetables, and an exercise program. My son is still able to eat a lot of food that I am happy to report he finds quite tasty. Currently he has shed 15 pounds and feels very proud of himself."*—MIKE GRADY, Toronto

In terms of fat consumption and obesity, it is important to remember that fats are significantly higher in the number of calories per gram in comparison to proteins and carbohydrates (9 calories per gram versus 4 calories per gram for carbohydrates and proteins). An excess intake of the wrong fats, such as saturated, hydrogenated, and partially hydrogenated fat, will lead to weight gain. These fats also make blood cells "stickier," resulting in fatty deposits and plaque buildup in the arterial walls. Processed and packaged foods will list saturated fats, partially hydrogenated fats, or hydrogenated fats as part of their ingredient list. When you see those words, move on—the product will only further complicate an obese child's condition. As mentioned in an earlier chapter, manufacturers do not have to list trans-fatty acids in their products. To avoid consumption of these dangerous fats, eliminate margarine, potato chips, and deep-fried foods such as french fries, onion rings, and doughnuts. It is also best to minimize saturated fats found in cheese, red meat, and butter when weight loss is desired

There are many tasty and healthy alternatives to these foods that will help children lose weight. Unless there is a genetic predisposition or hormonal problem that is causing the weight gain, a change in diet combined with physical activity always results in weight loss. As previously mentioned, I *never* recommend placing your children on a diet. It is far too restrictive and has an incredibly negative connotation for kids. I recommend focusing on healthy living by filling your kitchen cupboards and fridge with wholesome, fresh food such as whole grains, lean proteins, vegetables, and fruits. Instead of focusing on the perfect pant size (there is no such thing!) or what not to eat, emphasize positive attributes such as being strong and proud of their bodies whether they are short, tall, big, or small.

Instead of	Why not try
Margarine	Healthy nut butters, non-dairy or low-fat cream cheese, hummus (chickpea spread), or natural jams
French fries	Baked yam fries, lightly seasoned
Hamburgers, hot dogs	Veggie burger or hot dog
Potato chips, pretzels	Baked nachos or healthy granola mix
White cookies/breads	Whole grain cookies/breads made out of kamut, spelt, rye, or brown rice flour

IS BIGGER BETTER?

Realizing that the public has begun to equate more food with greater value, restaurants and fast-food chains all over North America have included extra food as incentives to lure patrons into their establishments. Free refills, all-you-can-eat buffets, and two-for-one pizzas are common marketing techniques used to attract consumers. The amount of food per serving has increased gradually over the years, causing people to eat more food without being aware of it. One of the most notorious food chains, McDonald's, has had a dramatic increase in the size of their best-selling french fries. According to *Nutrition Action Newsletter*:

> *In 1967, when McDonald's set up shop in Canada, it offered only one size of French fries, which weighed 84 grams and contained roughly 270 calories. Since then, the company's containers have exploded. While the 84 g fries are still on the menu (as a small), most people probably opt for the large (176 g and 560 calories) or super size (212 g and a whopping 680 calories).*[5]

Research clearly shows if people are served more food, they will overeat whether they are hungry or not. Most children no longer eat according to their appetite but rather unconsciously consume as much as they can, as quickly as they can. Instead of responding to their bodies' hunger cues, kids tend to wolf down excess calories of all the wrong foods. At first, in an attempt to maintain health, a child's digestive system will send subtle signals such as belching, burping, stomach aches, dark circles under the eyes, or skin rashes. If the digestive system continues to be overtaxed, more serious illnesses can develop such as clogging of arteries, poor response to insulin, and, of course, excess fat storage. In order to return to a state of health, it is important to make our children more aware of the amount they eat. If we look at nature, no other species suffers from obesity like the human species. Animals stop eating when they are satiated. Breast-feeding babies come off the nipple when their internal cue has signaled that they have had enough. I recommend showing your children what constitutes an appropriate amount of food. They should eat until they are sufficiently satiated, not stuffed. Have you ever noticed what it feels like when you overeat? You feel bloated, puffy, sluggish, irritable, and eager for the feeling to pass. Kids experience the same feelings. When children overeat, they become so lethargic that they are more inclined to plop themselves in front of a television or video than to participate in a mental or physical activity. Helping our children become more aware of the amount of food they are eating is one of the first steps we can take to prevent the battle of the bulge. Remember, most modern day diseases in North America are a result of overindulgence, not underindulgence. Perpetual overeating is one of the quickest roads to sickness and disease.

Thanks to the super sizing of portions, the total caloric content of a typical fast-food meal of cheeseburger, fries, and Coke has been hoisted to 1,340 calories from 680 calories. That is more than half a normal adult's recommended daily caloric consumption.

Many of us are no longer familiar with what constitutes a normal serving size. In reality, there are no standard serving sizes that are appropriate for each child. It is also not realistic to expect busy parents to take the time to measure every gram, cup, and serving their children eat at each meal (nor is it realistic to ask teenagers to do it for themselves). The key to awareness eating does not lie in tedious measurements but in paying attention to internal hunger cues. Start by encouraging your children to pay attention to when they are hungry, when they have overeaten, and when they are comfortably full from eating an appropriate amount of food. It is okay for your children to hear their stomachs grumbling once in a while. By doing so, you will teach them what true hunger is versus mindless eating and snacking. Although most of our parents did it, I do not recommend forcing children to clean their plates before being excused from the table. This practice forces children to eat when they are not hungry and further dissociates them from their true hunger cues. If children do not like what they are served at a meal, offer them a second or a third healthy alternative as an option. If those options are not appealing to them, they do not have to eat. Trust me, kids do not go hungry for long.

In addition to teaching children to focus on their hunger cues, encourage them to pay attention to how they feel after eating a specific food or snack. Do they want to have a nap after eating a plate of white spaghetti pasta? Do they get a runny nose after eating ice cream? Help them to communicate how the food they are eating makes them feel. Our bodies are always sending out subtle cues—we just have to start paying attention to them. After a meal or snack, symptoms such as sleepiness, hyperactivity, moodiness, an increase in mucous production, cravings, or sluggishness are not normal. If these symptoms occur, a child has either eaten too much, or has eaten the wrong food. Refer to Chapter 10 on allergies to help determine if your children suffer from food sensitivities and/or allergies.

Along with the increase in serving sizes, the pace of the family meal has also sped up. It is not uncommon for a family to gobble down a meal or snack within five minutes. There are even times when people are so rushed that they eat standing up! The best way to slow down your children's eating patterns is for the entire family to slow down. By doing so, you give the satiation signal the chance to register in the brain and will be inclined to eat less food. In the stomach there are stretch receptors that let the hypothalamus, the part of the brain that monitors hunger cues, know when it has received enough food. It takes about twenty minutes for the stretch receptors in the stomach to reach the brain. Most children shovel down their lunch or dinner, not allowing their full signal to click on. Without that signal, kids (and adults!) tend to over-eat. To make things worse, by shoveling in food and not chewing properly, children are sending undigested food particles down into their stomachs and small intestines as discussed in Chapter 3. Slowing down mealtime is one very effective method of battling the obesity problem. Encourage your children to chew, breathe, and focus on the various tastes, textures, and colors of the foods they are eating. To slow the pace at our table at mealtime, we play the "awareness eating game," which involves choosing an item on our plate that pleases us the most and sharing it with others. Whether it is the bright red color of a strawberry, the smell of fresh whole grain bread, or the perfectly ripened taste of an avocado, I am always amazed at how taking a moment to observe and be grateful for our food slows down our eating.

Kids in the United States ages seven to seventeen consume nearly twice as many calories when they eat at restaurants (average: 765 calories) than at home (average: 425 calories). Restaurant meals are also high in artery-clogging fat.[6]

The following tips are helpful in readjusting your children to the appropriate amount of food for their bodies:

- Try teaching your children to slow down at mealtime, using all five senses to enjoy their food. Sitting around a table together is an excellent time to review the day or express thoughts that are on their minds. Ideally, meals should last for at least half an hour.

- Encourage your kids to chew their food! Saliva has an enzyme called salivary amylase, which begins the breakdown of starchy foods.

- Select high-fiber foods such as fruits, vegetables, wholesome grains, and beans. These foods are very filling and create a satiated feeling.

- Avoid purchasing the super-sized foods offered at most establishments when dining out.

- Try eating more meals at home. Research clearly shows that people who dine out frequently at restaurants and fast-food chains are more likely to put on and store extra pounds.

- Do not allow your kids to mindlessly munch in front of the computer screen or TV. This habit will cause them to unconsciously overeat unhealthy treats.

- Eating is a good time to focus on just that—eating! Make mealtime a special, sacred time in your house to connect. Practise giving thanks for your food. If a formal grace before a meal does not feel comfortable, ask your children to choose their favorite things on their plates (based on color, smell, texture). This will help them appreciate the food they are about to receive.

DINING OUT

It is easy to monitor the amount children are eating at home, but what do you do when they go out? How do you prevent them from buying extra-large, super-sized, double-scoop, and double-patty burgers when they are hanging out at the mall, at a restaurant, or with friends at the local fast-food outlet? This is not so much of a concern for younger children who do not make independent food choices, but is for teens when obesity tends to develop. If your kids are old enough to purchase food and make their own food choices, they are old enough to understand the health consequences of overeating or eating the wrong foods. When dealing with an overweight child, always approach the subject in a sensitive, loving manner. Criticizing or critiquing them, even if out of concern, will only worsen the issue. It is best to emphasize shifting the entire family toward a state of optimal health and not on dieting to shed pounds. Once given the proper motivation and information, children will feel empowered to continue new, healthy eating habits inside and outside the home.

One of the biggest hurdles for parents is children's love of fast food. Fortunately, most fast-food chains have made considerable progress by introducing healthier alternatives to the standard hamburger, french fries, and Coke. I am still not a great advocate of eating fast foods because of the chemicals, oils, animal rights issues, etc., but often the situation is unavoidable. Items lower in fat and calories such as veggie burgers, veggie wraps, and salads are now available at fastfood chains across North America. These selections contain fewer calories and are lower in artery-clogging saturated fat. Make your children aware of these food alternatives and explain the benefits they have versus the traditional fast foods. Some other tricks to avoid excess calories when dining out are:

- Avoid ordering the large or extra-large sizes. Try ordering a medium or small and eat slowly to let your satiation signal kick in.

- Restaurants tend to pile on the cheese and cheese sauces on pizzas, pastas, bread, etc. Ask them to make your order light on the cheese or scoop off some of the excess yourself. Another healthier and less fattening alternative to a cream sauce is a delicious, red tomato sauce.

- Drink bottled water instead of pop or juice. Research shows that kids who drink sweetened soft drinks, iced tea, and fruit drinks are most likely to become obese.

- Avoid deep-fried foods such as french fries, calamari, onion rings, and doughnuts.

- Try to avoid overeating white, refined pasta.

- At a restaurant, skip the white bread and butter placed on the table at the beginning of the meal.

- Teach your children not to eat a large supper late at night. Research shows that eating more and later in the evening will lead to excess weight. As the light goes down, so does metabolic function.

- Try to include something fresh in every meal (fruits, vegetables, nuts, seeds, etc.) Not only are these foods filled with vital minerals and vegetables, they tend to fill you up faster.

- Stay away from cream-based soups filled with saturated fats and trans-fatty acids. Order soups that have a base of vegetable or chicken broth or are pureed.

If your child or teenager resists listening to you or other family members, consult an expert in the field. Nutritionist, dieticians, naturopaths, and various other health care practitioners can be just the person to kick-start the necessary changes for weight loss. When searching for a health care practitioner, try to find one with an integrative, holistic approach who will address the total needs (nutritional, physical, mental, spiritual, etc.) of your children. Children who are old enough may even be interested in doing some independent reading about their health care and bodies. There are many easy-to-understand books on the market that can provide a teenager with a more in-depth understanding of nutrition and its link to wellness. Teaching your children that they are major determinants of their own health is an invaluable lesson that will last a lifetime. Kids quickly realize that nothing is cooler or makes them feel better than liking their bodies and feeling healthy. Providing them with the nutritional knowledge to make their own smart food choices is one of the best ways to instill confidence.

Food Is a Right, Not a Privilege

It is a not uncommon for parents to use food to discipline younger children. Don't feel bad, there have been times when all of us have been ready to pull our hair out with our kids, nieces, nephews, or grandkids, and have turned to the closest sugary delight to soothe the situation. I frequently see parents in the grocery store using treats to ward off a child's potential temper tantrum. Why not? It is quick, easy, and usually does the job, right? I realize there are times when there are no other options, however, as a general rule, using food as a reward will only backfire on your children's health. This so-called positive reinforcement sends a message that good behavior results in receiving sweet-tasting goodies. This supports unhealthy eating habits.

Wholesome, good food is a child's birthright, not a privilege. There are many other effective methods for disciplining children without using food. When you do get the urge to use food bribes (and we all do!), make a conscious effort to use alternate reward systems such as the following:

- Reward good behavior with stickers. A great idea is to incorporate a calendar reward system. For example, a child receives a star sticker for every day of good behavior. A good run of stars (five to seven days) would result in a reward such as a special story, or a new book.

- If the opportunity presents itself and your children are not in the throes of a temper tantrum, try talking it out with them and helping them understand why you are asking them to do a specific chore, behave well, or use manners.

- Always keep a few books or small toys in your bag or purse for those difficult situations. It is much better to distract your children with a toy than to reward them with immune-suppressing sweets!

- Try honoring your children's likes and dislikes by having them choose how they spend family time. This can include a trip to an amusement park, the museum, their favorite park, etc.

- For older children and teenagers, positive incentives can include more time with friends, extra car time, or an extension on their curfew.

- If your children are often hungry, have small bags of fruit, vegetables, nuts, seeds, or granola available. Pack these snacks on a Sunday evening so you have a full stock to choose from for the week to come.

YOU GOTTA MOVE!

Regular exercise and a healthy diet go hand in hand for successful weight loss. Unfortunately, with our new generation of Nintendo kids, physical exercise is at an all-time low. In the United States in 1969, children watched an average of two hours of TV per day. This average increased to more than five hours per day in 1990. In one study, it was found that the incidence of obesity increased by 2 percent for every additional hour of television watched.[7]

Motivating an overweight child to start exercising can sometimes feel like an uphill battle. Not only are these youngsters lacking the energy required to become fit, most are also feeling insecure and embarrassed about their current physical state. They may feel uncomfortable about exercising in front of others or worried and hesitant to put on gym clothes. Being a kid can be hard enough without the added burden of feeling insecure about your pant size. Respect your children and do whatever it takes to implement an exercise regime that feels comfortable for them.

When starting an exercise program for children, choose an activity they enjoy. Whether it is walking the dog, joining a sports team, or dancing to music, as the Nike slogan states, "Just do it!" For children who are significantly overweight and/or out of shape, it is best to begin with a moderate to light exercise program. The key to success is to focus on motivation and enjoyment.

On average, children should exercise for at least one hour every day. Their intensity level should be determined by their current physical state and overall health. If necessary, speak to your primary health care practitioner about designing an exercise program specifically for your child. Although the chart on page 142 provides the number of calories burned for various exercises, I urge parents and kids not to focus on these values. I have provided this information only for reference.

Daily participation in high school physical education classes dropped from 42 percent in 1991 to 29 percent in 1999.[8]

When trying to lose weight, the key is to keep moving, apply healthy food principles outlined in earlier chapters, and be conscious of the amount of food eaten. By applying these three steps, your children will feel an enormous sense of satisfaction and accomplishment when the pounds start melting away. The following are suggestions for motivating your children to get moving:

- Take family walks or bike rides. Long hikes will help your children burn off excess calories while spending time with loved ones and nature.

- Limit the amount of television your children watch during the week. There is no reason for them to watch three or four hours of television or video per day. A good suggestion is to allow them an hour a day during the week for their favorite TV shows and two hours per day on weekends. Movies and videos can be saved for weekend treats.

- Set a good example for your children by exercising. The entire family can play a game of basketball, join the family community center, or turn on music and dance when cleaning the dishes!

- Sign up your children for various team sports that they enjoy. Dance, soccer, hockey, swimming lessons, and karate are all excellent options.

- Teenagers may be interested in working out on their own. Most gyms now offer a free initial personal training session that can help them get started.

- Remove all televisions and computers from your children's bedrooms.

The following table shows the number of calories burned when each exercise is done for twenty minutes:

Activities and Number of Calories Burned

Activity	Calories
Light walking	80
Dancing	120
Running	90
Cycling	160
Swimming	100
Skipping	100
Weights	140
Skiing	130

There is not much difference in calories burned in walking (80) versus running (90). Getting your children to participate in an after-dinner walk is almost as effective as a light jog or run.

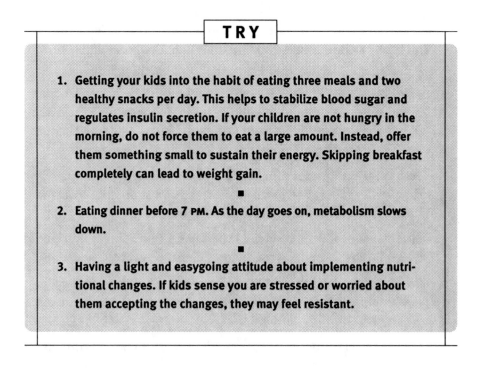

TRY

1. Getting your kids into the habit of eating three meals and two healthy snacks per day. This helps to stabilize blood sugar and regulates insulin secretion. If your children are not hungry in the morning, do not force them to eat a large amount. Instead, offer them something small to sustain their energy. Skipping breakfast completely can lead to weight gain.

   ■

2. Eating dinner before 7 PM. As the day goes on, metabolism slows down.

   ■

3. Having a light and easygoing attitude about implementing nutritional changes. If kids sense you are stressed or worried about them accepting the changes, they may feel resistant.

■

4. Incorporating a healthy goodie box that contains nutritious snacks such as nuts, seeds, dried fruits, seasoned soy nuts, baked chips, and homemade healthier cookies.

■

5. Avoiding disciplining with food. If your children are overweight, do not offer them food as consolation. Offer them a hug, your words of comfort, and lots of love.

NOTES

1 "Diet and Health—10 Mega-trends," *Nutrition Action Newsletter* 28 (January/February 2001).

2 www.aacap.org

3 M. Murray, *Diabetes and Hypoglycemia* (Rocklin, CA: Prima Health, 1994).

4 my.webmd.com

5 "Diet and Health—10 Mega-trends," *Nutrition Action Newsletter* 28 (January/February 2001).

6 *Nutrition Action Health Letter*, Canadian Edition 28(9) (November 2001).

7 W.H. Dietz and S.L. Gortmaker, "Do We Fatten Our Children at the Television Set? Obesity and Television Viewing in Children and Adolescents" *Paediatrics* 75, 1985. 807–812.

8 www.cdc.gov

CHAPTER 9

Attention Deficit Hyperactivity Disorder and Attention Deficit Disorder

I N ONE CLASSROOM, a child, unable to contain himself, jumps out of his seat, blurting out the answers to questions, causing quite the disruption for fellow students and the teacher. Another child, fidgeting with her hands, does not respond to her mother when asked repeatedly to empty the dishwasher. A third child constantly loses her glasses, forgets her school assignments, and continually daydreams. What do these three children have in common? They have all been diagnosed with the most common behavioral disorder—attention deficit hyperactivity disorder (ADHD).

DOES ADHD/ADD EXIST?

In the past twenty years, attention deficit hyperactivity disorder, also called attention deficit disorder (ADD), has become North America's leading childhood psychiatric disorder. The diagnoses of ADHD have grown from 500,000 in 1985 to between 5 and 7 million today.[1] The diagnosis of ADHD is relatively new—the criteria used to diagnose the disorder was first outlined by the American Psychological Association in 1980. Although the number of children diagnosed with this "brain disease" continues to rise, to date, no biological or organic origins for ADHD have been found. Some research studies attempted to link ADHD with a disruption or decrease in brain chemicals called neurotransmitters, however, there have been no sufficient physical findings yet to support this theory. In other words, there are no diagnostic testing procedures such as brain scans, blood analysis, or X rays that can decisively confirm or deny a diagnosis of ADHD. That said, ADHD is a real disorder that can have negative effects on a child's home, school, and social life. I recommend that parents and health care providers investigate all potential causes and/or triggers of the behavior prior to choosing drug therapy as their only course of action. Since diagnostic assessment lies strictly in criteria and description of various behaviors and is often made by untrained individuals, children run the risk of being wrongly diagnosed with ADHD and may be unnecessarily medicated. The incidence of ADHD elsewhere, such as Japan and Europe, is extremely low. If you or someone you know has a child who has been diagnosed with ADHD, it is in the best interest of that child to investigate all possible causes of the behavior and investigate the natural options available. Environmental irritants, school-based problems, food allergies, poor nutrition, and a deficiency in vital fats and minerals are all areas that should be explored.

WHAT ARE THE CRITERIA?

ADHD is diagnosed four times more frequently in boys than in girls and can also occur in adults. Diagnoses are made when a child's behavior is consistent with various criteria outlined in the *Diagnostic and Statistical Manual of Mental Disorders*, Fourth Edition (DSM-IV). The most common features associated with ADHD include:

- Distractibility (poor sustained attention to tasks)
- Impulsivity (impaired impulse control and delay of gratification)
- Hyperactivity (excessive activity and physical restlessness)

In order for a diagnosis to be made, behaviors must be excessive, long term, and pervasive. The behaviors must appear before the age of seven and continue for a minimum of six months. According to the DSM-IV, the following are common signs and symptoms of ADHD. Your child:

- Is restless
- Often does not seem to listen when spoken to directly
- Blurts out answers

- Fidgets with hands or feet
- Squirms
- Loses or forgets important things
- Talks excessively
- Has difficulty waiting in lines
- Does not follow through on instructions and fails to finish schoolwork
- Interrupts or intrudes on others
- Fails to give attention to details or makes careless mistakes in schoolwork
- Does not seem to listen when spoken to directly[2]

Of course, some of these behaviors seem like normal, everyday kid stuff, don't they? Generally, a diagnosis of ADHD occurs when a child's behavior has become disruptive to the school, social, or family environment. As mentioned, this is one of the most difficult disorders to diagnose and is subject to errors based on the analyst's interpretation and level of qualification.

Ritalin: A Pill for Every Ill?

The first line of treatment typically chosen by the allopathic model is a stimulant drug called Ritalin, or methylphenidate. Up to 90 percent of children diagnosed with ADHD receive a prescription for Ritalin. Ritalin is a class II controlled narcotic drug, which means it is in the same category as cocaine and potent barbiturates and opiates. Class II narcotic drugs have the greatest potential for addiction and abuse. Although Ritalin is effective in changing over 80 percent of children's behavior, its actual effect on a child's brain chemistry is not completely known. According to the *Physician's Desk Reference of Drug Side Effects* "the mode of action [of Ritalin] in man is not completely understood."[3] The drug appears to numb a child, suppressing all spontaneous behaviors such as curiosity, socialization, and play. Although, there are indeed specific cases where the use of Ritalin is warranted, for the most part, it does not address the root cause of the disorder, and has potentially dangerous side effects that every parent should be aware of.

Ritalin has been increasingly prescribed at an alarming rate in the pediatric population in the past several years. In 1996, the World Health

Organization warned that the overuse of Ritalin had reached dangerous proportions. According to Lawrence Diller, author of *Running on Ritalin*:

In 1997 alone, nearly five million people in the United States were prescribed Ritalin—most of them young children diagnosed with attention deficit disorder. Use of Ritalin, which is a stimulant related to amphetamine, has increased by 700 percent since 1990. And this phenomena appears to be uniquely American: 90 percent of the world's Ritalin is used in the United States.[4]

The two most common side effects of Ritalin are insomnia and loss of appetite. Unfortunately, not eating or sleeping are also the two quickest ways to suppress a healthy immune system. A child's system becomes at risk of suffering from a deficiency of calories, minerals, vitamins, and essential fats because of their lack of appetite. Insomnia also disrupts their learning capabilities with children feeling drowsy or falling asleep at school. To counteract the insomnia, doctors often prescribe a sedative for children to take at bedtime. Now we are really entering dangerous territory. How can it seem logical to put a child on an addictive, stimulant drug by day and a sedative by night? Surely there are other, more natural alternatives that should be explored first.

The US Army and the Coast Guard will not enlist anyone with a history of Ritalin use.

Ritalin has also been shown to create other psychological disturbances in children such as obsessive-compulsive disorder, aggression, and antisocial behavior. When this happens and a child's emotional state begins to collapse, it is not uncommon for them to be diagnosed with other emotional disorders such as schizophrenia or bipolar disorder that Ritalin has "unmasked." Eventually, these children can end up on four or five various medications, including neuroleptics, antidepressants, and antipsychotic medications.

Other known side effects of Ritalin are:

- Adverse cardiovascular effects
- Blood glucose changes
- Depression
- Disruption of growth hormone production

- Gastrointestinal upset
- Headache
- Increased blood pressure
- Irritability
- Jittery feelings
- Permanent change to brain chemistry
- Psychosis or paranoia
- Tics and repetitive movements

I have always found the idea of drug side effects rather comical. It is as if this term is used to dismiss the severity of other symptoms that may arise from taking a drug. *All alterations created by a drug that upset a body's normal functioning should be considered on an equal scale.* In my mind, there are no such things as side effects, only effects. Before putting children on any medication, all the effects and potential risks of a drug should be reviewed. Often this may take some investigative work of your own, but knowing this information is your right to.

Parents are often encouraged to allow their children to take a break from using Ritalin. For example, if a child's behavior is under control at home, it is recommended that the medication be stopped during the summer holidays or vacation in order to give the body a rest. In fact, while researching for this book, I came across a suggestion made by a well-known medical school that recommended, "If there are concerns about a child's growth (due to Ritalin), a drug holiday may be allowed for some catch up time to occur." This suggestion is totally illogical. If ADHD is a brain disease, why is a child's behavior acceptable at home but not in a classroom? Does the disease subside when a child is on vacation? It makes you wonder if medication is indeed the correct course of action to take.

> *The use of prescription stimulants such as Ritalin predisposes children to cocaine and nicotine abuse in young adulthood.*

There are situations where Ritalin is necessary, such as when a child is suicidal or when one has exhausted every other option. My concern is how quickly children are put on Ritalin, at the first sign of a behavioral problem. Parents, caregivers, and teachers should know that a diagnosis of ADHD does not always have to mean a lifetime of taking potent psychiatric drugs. As you will see in the following section, there are natural alternatives available. Discuss alternatives to Ritalin or other stimulants with your children's doctor. That said, do not take your children off Ritalin without speaking to your doctor. Withdrawal from psychiatric drugs can have adverse effects and must be done gradually under medical supervision.

NATURAL APPROACHES TO ADHD

When addressing an ADHD child's needs, an integrative, therapeutic approach involving several professionals often has the best outcome. For example, the physician's role is to diagnose and provide the appropriate medications, the mental health professional provides supportive counseling and coping strategies for parents, and the teacher provides parents with feedback about the effectiveness of the stimulant on classroom behavior. Curiously, conventional treatment of ADHD rarely mentions the role of nutrition and supplements as part of a complete integrative and less intrusive approach. In the medical community, the nutritional benefits for children suffering from ADHD are deemed unscientific and anecdotal at best. However, recent research suggests that nutrition plays an extremely important role in the treatment and prevention of ADHD. Studies show that the blood-brain barrier and the gut wall in ADHD children are more permeable, allowing in toxins such as metals, solvents, pesticides, PCBs, alcohol, and drugs.[5]

With the dramatic rise in the number of children diagnosed with this disorder, it is wise to examine what elements have changed in the past twenty years that may be contributing to the rise in ADHD. Environmental pollution is at an all-time high, preservatives and dyes are pervasive in our foods, and the overall quality of children's nutrition has dropped. According to a recent article in *alive* magazine:

> *The global increase in chemicals is staggering. In the US alone, synthetic organic chemical production rose from a few billion pounds a year in 1945, to 163 billion pounds a year in 1985. Chlorine production rose from three to 12 billion pounds a year between 1930 and 1985. These chemicals include all known PCBs, DDTs, 2, 4-Ds, polyvinyl chloride, gasoline byproducts and heavy metals such as lead, aluminum, cadmium and mercury.*[6]

Our children are bombarded with toxins that previous generations were not exposed to. Cancer rates in kids are up, obesity and related disease processes are escalating, and behavioral disorders also appear to be on the rise. A holistic approach to ADHD involves addressing classroom issues, disciplining techniques, spending quality time with your children, removing harmful toxins from their diet, and replacing them with healing foods and supplements. Instead of choosing stimulant drugs such as Ritalin as your first treatment option, make it your last resort. Exhaust all natural and less invasive treatments that will benefit your children's health in the future. Drugs should be reserved for the most severe cases or as a last resort when all other alternatives have failed.

Parents often ask why, if two children are eating the same diet, why does one develop ADHD and another does not? As mentioned earlier, everyone is biochemically different. One person's body processes food, thoughts, and emotions differently than the next. It is similar to one child excelling in math and the other becoming the next Picasso. In terms of health, there are definitely inexplicable individual differences that make certain children more sensitive to environmental toxins and foods. Illness manifests differently from child to child. Sally may develop a rash or throat infection from eating too many sweets, while Billy may act out at home or in the classroom. A pollutant, virus, bacteria, or food will usually affect a child's weakest link. Often it is the intestinal system, which creates systemic symptoms throughout the body. The importance of intestinal health only lends more support to shifting children back to a wholesome diet to preserve optimal health.

There is no one solution for kids with ADHD. As mentioned, there can be many triggers, including heavy metal toxicities, nutritional deficiencies, birth defects, genetic abnormalities, hormonal disturbances, and food and chemical allergies. When parents first make changes to their children's diet, they may have to try several options before clearly identifying what works and what does not. Don't be discouraged—the trial and errors are worth the effort if they can stabilize a child's behavior naturally and without drugs.

The following are the nutritional causes that have been associated with ADHD:

- Food additives, dyes, and preservatives
- Food allergies

- Deficiency in omega-3 fatty acid and ingestion of too many "funny fats"
- Refined sugars and carbohydrates
- Antibiotics and yeast
- Deficiency of various minerals and vitamins
- Heavy metal toxicity

Eliminating Food Additives

The idea that food can have an effect on behavior became popularized in the early 1970s due to the research conducted by Benjamin Feingold, MD, pediatrician and allergist. Dr. Feingold advocated a diet free of salicylates (chemicals similar to aspirin that are found in a wide variety of foods), food coloring, and artificial flavoring to reduce hyperactive behavior in children. In his research, Dr. Feingold reported improvement in behavior in approximately 32–60 percent of all children tested. Dr. Feingold's research and results have been a topic hotly debated in the medical world. Follow-up research on the Feingold diet showed mixed reports; some studies have reproduced Feingold's results on behavior, while others showed that the Feingold diet has little or no effect.

Feingold's food elimination trials are often recommended in two stages. Stage I includes removing all food additives including food dyes, synthetic flavorings, BHT, BHA, benzoates, MSG, nitrates, and nitrites. If behavior does not improve, stage II involves eliminating all foods containing salicylates including:

- Almonds
- Apples
- Apricots
- Aspirin
- Berries (all)
- Cherries
- Cider and cider vinegar
- Cloves
- Coffee
- Cucumbers
- Currants
- Grapes
- Nectarines
- Oranges
- Peaches
- Pickles
- Plums
- Prunes
- Raisins
- Tangerines
- Tea
- Tomatoes
- Vinegar
- Wine

After a favorable response has been observed for four to six weeks, the foods eliminated in stage II can be reintroduced one at a time. Because most fruits and vegetables containing vitamin C are eliminated from the diet in stage II, supplementation may be necessary.[7] According to Dr. Feingold, children under the age of six respond to the diet within one week, while children over the age of six may need to follow the diet for two to six weeks to achieve results. For more information about Dr. Feingold's diet, visit www.feingold.org.

Identifying Food Allergies

The following chapter details specifics on food allergies, methods to determine if your children suffer from food allergies, and the natural means to control them. The take home point for this chapter is to understand that food allergies and/or sensitivities can be responsible for behavioral changes in children and should be considered in treatment. The most common allergic foods for children include dairy products, wheat, citrus fruits, chocolate, tomatoes, soy, eggs, and corn. If food allergies are suspected, eliminate these common allergic foods to see if there is a change in behavior. A potential food trigger should be eliminated for at least two weeks before any difference is discernible.

Supplementing with Omega-3

Omega-3 essential fatty acids provide the building blocks necessary for the healthy development of neurological tissues and proper brain function. Current research indicates that children who suffer from ADHD may be deficient in linolenic acid (omega-3) and its derivative, DHA. It appears that boys require more omega-3 than girls, which may be one of the reasons why ADHD is more prevalent in the younger male population. Omega 3-deficiency syndrome is a widespread problem affecting adults and children throughout North America. Currently, approximately 20 percent of all people in the United States are so deficient in omega-3 that none can be detected in their blood. Consider the following studies:

- Hyperactive children were found to have lower levels of key fatty acids in their blood than normal children. The hyperactive kids were more likely to report symptoms of omega-3 deficiency such as thirst, dry hair and skin, and were also more likely to have asthma and ear infections.[8]

- A study at Purdue University is leaning toward the conclusion that ADHD is due to a deficiency of DHA. The researchers also found that children with ADHD were breast-fed far less often as infants than were children without ADHD. Breast milk is an excellent source of DHA.[9]

- Studies with non-human primates and human newborns indicate that DHA (omega-3) is essential for the normal functional development of the retina and the brain, particularly in premature infants. Because omega-3 fatty acids are essential in growth and development throughout the life cycle, they should be included in the diet of all humans.[10]

All cellular membranes in the body and synaptic endings of neurons (brain cells) in the brain require DHA. Without DHA, nerve transmissions do not function properly. The influx of chemically altered fats in the form of partially hydrogenated or hydrogenated oils compounds the omega-3 problem. As was outlined in Chapter 6 on fats, the shape of these oils has been altered and therefore they no longer fit properly into cell receptors. Research shows that hydrogenated and partially hydrogenated oils can create cellular damage and upset the flow of nervous system signals that regulate behavior, thereby worsening an already existing omega-3 deficiency. Refined and processed products such as crackers, chips, pretzels, commercial peanut butter, salad dressings, and microwave popcorn are potential sources of funny fats.

With the decreased quality of food sources available today, it is very hard to consume a sufficient amount of omega-3 essential fatty acids from your diet. To ensure that your children are receiving a sufficient amount of omega-3, purchase a fish oil or flaxseed oil from a health food store. Give them 1 teaspoon of fish oil or flaxseed oil per day. To disguise the oil, put it in a juice or shake. Flaxseed oil can also be used for salad dressings, marinade on top of vegetables, and popcorn topping. Never heat these oils—doing so can create dangerous alterations in their chemical structure that can be harmful to health. If your children find the oil in their juice or shake unpalatable and are old enough to swallow a capsule without difficulty, omega-3 supplements are also available in capsule form (refer to Appendix IV). Store your flax and fish oil in the refrigerator and check the label to see if your omega-3 capsules need to be refrigerated.

Omega-3 deficiencies in children respond very quickly (within a month) to supplementation. Keep a close eye on changes in your children's behavior and improvements in symptoms consistent with an omega-3 deficiency such as:

- Improvement in dryness of skin or other skin conditions such as eczema
- Less thirst
- Hair appears to have more luster and shine
- Allergies have lessened or subsided
- Asthma attacks have lessened in severity
- Inflammatory responses improve
- Gastrointestinal symptoms subside
- Behavior improves

If your children do not respond to omega-3 supplementation with flaxseed oil, their digestive systems may not have the capacity to break down omega-3 into its absorbable derivative DHA. If this is the case, try using fish oils or purchasing a supplement that contains a high percentage of absorbable DHA.

Eliminating Refined Sugars and Carbohydrates

Although most research studies have not yet found a scientific link between hyperactivity and white sugar and carbohydrate consumption, many parents would strongly disagree. To some, the dramatic changes in their children's behavior after eating a sugary delight is undeniable. We have all seen children who bounce off the walls after eating a big piece of birthday cake. It is obvious that these children are experiencing a sugar high. Despite the lack of proper research into this area, there is reason to believe that sugar is indeed a trigger of behavioral changes in a child. As explained in Chapter 4 on carbohydrates, refined sugars and carbohydrates enter the bloodstream at a rapid rate, resulting in an elevation of blood sugar. Following the rapid rise in blood sugar, and in an attempt to restore balance, the body will secrete the hormone insulin to lower blood sugar levels. When blood sugar levels fall too low, a state known as reactive hypoglycemia (low blood sugar) occurs. Reactive hypoglycemia can create symptoms of brain fog, moodiness, hyperactivity, inability to pay attention, headaches, psychological disturbances, and irritability. It is possible that symptoms diagnosed as ADHD may be the result of fluctuations in a child's blood sugar. Hold on—there is more to this vicious cycle. Since a hypoglycemic state is not an ideal state for the body to be in, the body attempts to maintain balance by recruiting the help of the adrenal glands (two small glands that sit on top of the kidneys). The adrenal glands are triggered to secrete a hormone called adrenaline to kick-start a feeling of energy in the body. Increased adrenaline secretion in kids can result in a hyperactive state, thus continuing the cycle of mood swings.

If your children suffer from ADHD or other behavioral problems, I recommend strictly eliminating sugar and refined carbohydrates for a two-week period to monitor the effects. Substitute with the healthier grains and sugars that are outlined in Chapter 4.

Eliminating Antibiotics and Yeast

Sooner or later, most children will be on a dose of antibiotics for an ear or bronchial infection. After the common cold, ear infections are the most common illness diagnosed in children. In fact, one-third of all children will have three or more ear infections by the time they reach their third birthday. According to Murray and Pizzorno, authors of *The Encyclopaedia of Natural Medicine*, "frequent ear infections and antibiotic use are associated with a greater likelihood of developing ADD." As mentioned in a previous chapter, although antibiotics are useful at certain times for killing off the bad bacteria, they also kill off the good bacteria (the microflora) that naturally exist in our intestinal tract. Overuse of broad-spectrum antibiotics in children compromises the microflora, which promotes the overgrowth of yeast, also known as candida albicans. The proliferation of yeast in the intestinal lining can create little holes or gaps in the intestinal wall. These small openings can create leaky gut syndrome where undigested proteins, carbohydrates, and toxins can leak through. When this occurs, an immune response is triggered in the body that can result in a myriad of symptoms. It is possible that a child's aggressive or unmanageable behavior diagnosed as ADHD may in fact be caused by an unhealthy digestive system and an overgrowth of yeast. Classic symptoms consistent with an overgrowth of yeast are:

- Abdominal gas and bloating
- Anxiety/panic attacks
- Brain fog
- Constipation
- Cravings for sugar and sweets
- Headaches
- Inability to concentrate
- Irritability
- Lethargy
- Mental confusion
- Mood swings
- Tonsillitis/recurrent strep throat
- Weight gain

An overgrowth of yeast and its link to ADHD is not something that is commonly discussed in the allopathic model. In fact, most medical doctors have never been taught about the side effects of an overgrowth of yeast and may think you are a little wacky if you suggest this as a possibility. However, there are medical doctors well versed in holistic medicine, naturopaths, and nutritionists who are quite familiar with the toxic effects of yeast. Consulting an experienced practitioner can be of great help in restoring your children's intestinal health.

If you suspect your children may be suffering from an overgrowth of yeast, start by eliminating all refined carbohydrates and sugars. Yeast loves to grow in the environment that these foods provide. If your children are over the age of two, supplement their diet with the good bacteria called lactobacillus acidophilus. If they are under the age of two, their diet can be supplemented with lactobacillus bifidus. Both of these supplements increase the growth of the friendly bacteria necessary for intestinal health, leaving little room for yeast to grow. Acidophilus and bifidus are available in capsule or powder form in most health food stores. It is best to take these supplements on an empty stomach. If your children find this too difficult, the supplement can be mixed into their food, water, or juice. Acidophilus and bifidus must be stored in the fridge.

Yeast can be difficult to get rid of and may initially require what feels like a very restrictive dietary change and a multitude of supplements. Although it will take a lot of effort in the beginning, it is always best to deal with an overgrowth of yeast at the earliest age possible. When children first change to a candida-free diet and take proper supplements, the yeast will die off. When this occurs, symptoms sometimes become worse. Do not be alarmed if your children's behavior or other physical symptoms get worse before they get better. If the infection is quite severe and is not responding to the above changes recommended, speak to your doctor about the possibility of using the drug Nystatin. Nystatin is a powerful prescription drug that works as an intestinal antiseptic against yeast. For more detailed information on a yeast-free diet, the book *The Yeast Connection* by William Crook and Cynthia Crook is an excellent resource.

Supplementing with Minerals and Vitamins

The brain relies on minerals and vitamins to function at an optimal state. Because there are so many nutrient-void foods, kids are often deficient in various minerals and vitamins. For example, iron deficiency is the most common mineral deficiency in North American children today. It is associated with lethargy, inattentiveness, decreased attention span, and decreased persistence. Other mineral deficiencies found in children with ADHD and learning disorders are copper, zinc, calcium, and magnesium. If a child is deficient in certain minerals and vitamins, there are two possibilities:

1. Either the deficiencies are due to a lack of proper nutritional intake in their diet, or
2. are due to poor digestion and absorption.

If the mineral deficiency is due to poor digestion and absorption, cleaning up the digestive system with healing herbs, supplements, "good bacteria," and food sources will greatly benefit a child. If children are deficient in various minerals because of poor intake and are suffering from ADHD, I recommend a high-quality multivitamin/multimineral complex to act as a nutritional safety net. Vitamins and minerals should never be used as a replacement for healthy eating; rather, they should complement a good diet. Research clearly shows that supplementation can improve a child's performance at school. Children should take their vitamins with food for better overall absorption of the fat-soluble vitamins A, D, E, and K. Have them take their vitamins at the same time every day (i.e., with breakfast) to get into the habit of supplementing daily. Most health food stores carry pediatric powdered or liquid supplements if your children have difficulty swallowing pills.

Eliminating Heavy Metal Toxins

Increased levels of lead, cadmium, copper, and mercury have all been linked to learning disorders and behavioral changes in children. A hair analysis is one test to help determine whether or not these heavy metals have accumulated in your children's systems. A whole food diet, supplementation with a high-quality multimineral/multivitamin, and improving gastrointestinal health are all effective techniques for reducing the levels of heavy metals in the body.

THINK TWICE

Prior to accepting a diagnosis of ADHD, I recommend visiting more than one health care professional. It is important to be cautious when diagnosing children with behavioral problems. Children internalize everything, especially when the message comes from mom or dad. When they are told that their behavior is the problem and medication is the solution, does this shift the blame onto their tiny shoulders? Studies show that children with ADHD are more predisposed to crime, poor school grades, and drug addiction. Is this the result of a true genetic disorder, the medications they have been taking, or is there an element of self-fulfilling prophecy? Of course, there are no studies or research available to substantiate the psychological effects of a diagnosis on children, but it is an area that should be considered. If your children really do suffer from a behavioral disorder, assure them that you and the entire family will do whatever it takes to help. It is very easy to become frustrated and angry when children continually act out and do not pay attention, but, whenever possible, try to focus on nurturing them with love, hugs, and discipline. It is vital not to give these kids the message that they are bad and that the medication will make them good. Try to remember that their behavior does not define their essence; it is a challenge to deal with. Changes in behavior are more likely to occur with positive classroom changes, healthy nutrition, proper supplementation, psychological counseling, and appropriate disciplining techniques.

TRY

1. Eliminating all refined sugars and carbohydrates from your children's diet. Switch them to a diet of whole grains, fruits, vegetables, and fish.

   ■

2. Avoiding eating at fast-food restaurants. These foods are loaded with chemicals and preservatives that can create dramatic mood changes in children.

   ■

3. Getting your children to drink a lot of water to flush their system. Avoid sugary juices and caffeinated beverages.

   ■

4. Eliminating all dyed foods from your children's diet (such as red licorice, icing, candy, etc.). Start packing homemade, healthier snacks when going to the movies.

   ■

5. Advising grandparents, caregivers, and other people who take care of your children that you are eliminating food preservatives and sugar from your children's diet. Instruct them *not* to give your children products that contain these ingredients.

NOTES

1 http://www.adhdfraud.org/

2 *The Diagnostic and Statistical Manual of Mental Disorder*, 4th edition.

3 www.drday.com

4 L. Diller, *Running on Ritalin* (New York: Bantam Books, 1998).

5 S. Whillier, *Nutritional Pathology and the Health Care of the Future* (Richmond Hill: CSNN Publishing, 1999).

6 Dr. J. Krop, "Toxic Treating Bodies with Environmental Medicine," *alive* magazine 231 (January 2002).

7 http://www.hacsg.org.uk/index.html

8 L.J. Stevens et al., "Essential Fatty Acid Metabolism in Boys with Attention-Deficit Hyperactivity Disorder," *American Journal of Clinical Nutrition* 62 4 (October 1995): 761–768.

9 J.R. Burgess et al., "Long-Chain Polyunsaturated Fatty Acids in Children with Attention Deficit Hyperactivity Disorder," *American Journal of Clinical Nutrition* 71 (January 2000): 321S–330S.

10 A. Simopoulos, "Omega-3 Fatty Acids in Health and Disease and in Growth and Development," *American Journal of Clinical Nutrition* 54 (1991): 438–463.

CHAPTER 10

Allergies

WHY IS IT that a food will have no effect on one child but can cause ear infections, bronchial spasms, or hives in another? The secret may lie in your children's diet. Certain foods that are nutritious for one child can wreak histamine havoc on the system of another, causing uncomfortable and chronic allergic reactions.

Remember the complexities of biochemical individuality—an allergy or sensitivity will manifest itself differently from child to child. If your children suffer from any of the signs and symptoms listed below, it is wise to start paying attention to their diet and the timing of their symptoms. An effective way to pinpoint the potential food trigger is to record a seven-day food diary of everything eaten by your children and any correlating symptoms. It is important to record timing of symptoms as well because allergic responses may take anywhere from hours to days to manifest. The most common signs and symptoms related to food allergies and food sensitivities in children are:

- Allergic shiners (puffiness or dark circles under the eyes)
- Anxiety
- Asthma
- Attention deficit disorder
- Bed-wetting
- Bronchial infections
- Colic
- Constipation
- Crohn's or colitis
- Diarrhea
- Ear infections
- Eczema
- Frequent infections
- Hyperactivity
- Irritable bowel syndrome
- Obesity or excess weight
- Rashes
- Runny nose
- Spitting up in infants
- Vomiting

Currently, medical doctors do not receive sufficient training on the adverse effects of food allergies and sensitivities on children's health. This is an area rarely addressed during visits to a pediatrician. When allergies are investigated, the standard diagnostic tool used is the scratch test or intradermal test. A small dose of allergens is injected under the skin. The doctor then notes if a reaction to the allergen occurs such as a wheal or a small bubble that may be red or inflamed. While this test is a good indicator of an immediate skin reaction to environmental allergies such as dust and mold, it does not deal with the complexity of food allergies and intolerances. If the body is sensitive to a certain food, widespread negative symptoms can be produced affecting the intestinal tract, respiratory system, skin, and other organs. In this chapter you will learn how to identify signs and symptoms of food allergies, diagnostics that are available to detect food sensitivities, and natural methods to halt allergies and return even the most allergic child back to a state of health. Although certain factors can predispose a child to developing food allergies such as genetics (one or both parents are allergy sufferers), if the core problem is linked to nutritional deficiencies and/or food reactions, there are many steps that can be taken. With proper supplementation and a wholesome diet, your children will not need antihistamine drugs, corticosteroids, or allergy shots for life.

Food allergies and other adverse reactions to food are now reported in about 25 percent of young children.[1]

When determining food allergies, there are two categories that should be examined:

1. Foods that are so toxic to the body that their effect on health is always negative. These non-foods are coffee, white sugar, aspartame, preservatives, and food dyes. They create an anti-nutrient and draining effect on a child's system and should be kept to a minimum in all diets. The body will always perceive these foods and preservatives as invaders and create a negative reaction.

2. The second category of food is nutritious to most, but has been identified as the most common allergy triggers in children. They are dairy products, wheat, citrus fruits, chocolate, tomatoes, soy, eggs, and corn.

WHAT IS AN ALLERGY?

There is great debate among the medical community regarding the true definition of the word "allergy." Physiologically, an allergic response or sensitivity to a food occurs when the body, for various reasons, perceives an otherwise harmless food as a dangerous invader. Similar to a bacteria or virus, the food invader triggers an outpouring of antibodies (specifically immunoglobins IgE or IgG) whose main goal is to eliminate the invader through various responses such as respiratory (asthma), digestive (vomiting or diarrhea), or through the skin (eczema). When an allergic response is immediate, it involves the excess production of immunoglobin IgE, which triggers the release of histamine from cells. A release of histamine in the body results in symptoms such as wheezing, skin rashes, and excess mucous production.

In contrast to immediate reactions, food intolerances (also called food sensitivities) produce signs and symptoms that are variable and often delayed. It appears that the release of immunoglobins IgG is responsible for the development of food sensitivities. Food sensitivities can develop for reasons such as poor digestive health, overconsumption of anti-nutrient foods, and lack of variety in the diet. For example, children who eat refined wheat products over and over again may eventually become intolerant to wheat and suffer from chronic respiratory infections. Because food intolerances/sensitivities are not as obvious, they are often called the hidden problem. As a general rule, if your children are eating the right foods for their bodies, an adverse response, even as mild as a runny nose, following an ice cream cone should not occur. The good news is that with proper nutrition, elimination diets, and supplement therapy, food intolerances can often be eliminated. In this chapter, I will be using the terms food intolerance and food sensitivity interchangeably.

IMMEDIATE VERSUS DELAYED RESPONSE

As mentioned, reaction to a food can be immediate or delayed. In a few cases, immediate reactions can be quite severe and are classified as an anaphylactic allergy. For example, an anaphylactic reaction occurs when a child's breathing is immediately compromised after eating a peanut. Anaphylactic reactions should be taken very seriously as they are life-threatening. Strict avoidance of the food must be adhered to. Anaphylactic allergies are considered fixed allergies that cannot be changed. Parents and caregivers usually know if a child suffers from an anaphylactic allergy and therefore take the necessary precautions such as reading labels, avoiding restaurants that do not list their ingredients, and carrying an EpiPen (a shot of epinephrine injected into the skin) in case of emergency. Only 1 percent of all children have anaphylactic allergies. The second type of allergic reaction is a delayed response that can occur hours and even days after eating a particular food. I will refer to this type of reaction as a food intolerance or food sensitivity. For example, Billy, who is unknowingly allergic to dairy, may develop an ear infection two days after eating a vanilla ice cream cone. The doctor will put Billy on his third round of antibiotics that year. Unfortunately, antibiotics will kill off the good bacteria in the gut, allowing for the overgrowth of unhealthy microbes such as yeast, further aggravating the condition. Parents and children often get trapped in this vicious cycle. If steps are not taken to remove the dairy from Billy's diet and restore proper bowel health, the ear infection is likely to recur. If Billy's intolerance to dairy is not investigated and addressed, he runs the risk of being placed on more antibiotics and may even face surgical intervention. Detecting food sensitivities in a child can feel like looking for a needle in a haystack. However, with the guidance of a well-trained health care practitioner and the proper information, the food culprit can be identified and removed.

> *Studies indicate that if one parent suffers from a respiratory allergy, a child has a 30–50 percent chance of developing an allergy. If both parents suffer from respiratory allergies, there is a 60–80 percent chance of a child developing an allergy.*

If symptoms do occur following the ingestion of certain foods, these are some possible causes:

- A child has eaten an excessive amount of the same type of food.

- A child is suffering from poor digestive health because of stress or frequent use of broad-spectrum antibiotics, pesticides, preservatives, or food dyes.

- A child has eaten too much food and has overloaded his or her system.

- The immune system is compromised.

- There is a decreased production in stomach acid (Hcl) or other digestive enzymes.

- There is a predisposition to a heightened allergic response because of genetics.

GETTING TO THE BOTTOM OF IT!

When it comes to children's food intolerances, parents are often left to do their own homework. The current medical approach used to deal with allergies is to suppress the body's natural immune response. The two types of drugs most commonly used are antihistamines to stop histamine release, and corticosteroids to halt inflammation. These medications are very effective at masking symptoms, but can be problematic when used for lengthy periods. Often chronic use of these medications can result in a *rebound effect* when the medication is eventually stopped. Have you ever wondered why your allergic symptoms seem to become worse when you stop taking a certain drug? This is a classic example of the rebound effect. Because the body's natural response has been suppressed, when given the opportunity, it responds with more severe symptoms. These medications are appropriate in certain cases, however, their long-term use can cause even more problems and side effects. Here are the standard treatment options used by the allopathic model of medicine:

- **Antihistamines:** Treat the symptoms by suppressing the body's histamine response

- **Decongestants:** Reduce congestion

- **Desensitization shots:** Allergy shots

- **Laser surgery:** Use of laser to vaporize mucous-forming nasal tissue

- **Steroid nasal sprays:** Long-term effect unknown

Integrative medicine, on the other hand, takes a different approach to allergies by investigating why the body is triggering a heightened immune reaction to an otherwise harmless food. Does the child suffer from poor digestion? Poor absorption? Is the child eating the same foods over and over again? There are several tests available to help determine if food allergies are the cause of your children's illness or infections. Some of the tests available are very accurate, and others are rather crude. I recommend finding a health care practitioner who uses a combination of various diagnostic procedures.

The following tests are listed from the most to the least accurate in determining food allergies. To have some of these tests or trials done, you will likely have to visit an "alternative" health care practitioner.

Elimination/Rotation Diets

An elimination diet involves removing the suspected food allergens from the diet and switching to a hypoallergenic diet. The foods that should be eliminated first are the non-foods (such as white sugar, aspartame, caffeine, etc.) and the most common food irritants (such as dairy, wheat, gluten, corn, soy, eggs, citrus fruits, chocolate, and tomatoes). Hypoallergenic diets include foods such as lamb, chicken, potatoes, brown rice, apples, bananas, broccoli, cabbage, and Brussel sprouts. These foods are fairly bland and difficult to implement for young children, but are the most effective approach. Allergic foods should be eliminated one by one for at least three weeks before any differences will be noticeable. (In addition to an elimination diet, please refer to the section below on supplements that can help lessen and eliminate the allergic response.)

During the initial stages of an elimination diet, it is not uncommon for children's allergy symptoms or food cravings to temporarily worsen. This is normal and the body's way of attempting to restore biochemical balance. To reduce this effect, make sure they consume an abundant amount of fresh, filtered water and/or supplement with pediatric chewable vitamin C tablets (use only if a child is old enough to thoroughly chew food). If diarrhea occurs when vitamin C is given, cut the dosage in half. If diarrhea persists, stop the vitamin C supplementation. It is also common for children to lose a small amount of weight in the initial stage of an elimination diet. This is usually the loss of water that was once retained by eating the allergic food. As long as their diet maintains the necessary amount of calories for their size, their optimal weight will balance out.

Once a child's digestive system has been cleaned up, the potential food culprit may be slowly reintroduced three weeks following its removal to test for a reaction. When first reintroducing the food, give only a small amount. If no reaction occurs, that particular food may be included in the diet, but only on a rotational basis (no more than once every four days). In other words, if a child consumes soy on Monday, it should not be eaten again until Friday. If the food is once again eaten in excess, chances are the child will again develop intolerance to it. *Remember, the foods we eat the most, and the foods we crave are usually the ones that we are most allergic or sensitive to.* If a reaction does occur following the reintroduction of a specific food, a child's system is either not healthy enough to digest it properly, or the child's body will never be able to accept that particular food. For example, certain children will never be able to eat dairy products without having a negative respiratory response. This type of food allergy is fixed and the food must always be avoided. Alternatively, you can wait for another three weeks and retest the body's response. However, if a child suffers from anaphylactic allergies, never reintroduce allergic foods. When implementing an elimination/rotation diet, it is best to do so under the supervision of a health care practitioner experienced in the area of food sensitivities such as a naturopath or nutritionist.

Elimination/rotation diets are extremely effective in determining food allergies and renewing digestive health. Although this diet is time-consuming and requires a parent's dedication, it is well worth the effort.

Blood Analysis: The ELISA Test

The ELISA blood analysis measures the presence of antibodies and white blood cell reactions to certain foods. This test can measure immediate allergic reactions (IgE) and/or delayed hidden allergies (IgG). It can eliminate the need for lengthy and tedious elimination/rotation diets, which can be difficult to implement in children. The drawback is that it is fairly costly ($120–$1,200) and is not typically ordered by most medical doctors. For more information on the ELISA test, visit Great Smokies Diagnostic Laboratory at www.gsdl.com.

Muscle Testing

Muscle testing is an excellent technique to determine food allergies. The concept of muscle testing is based on the Chinese meridian system and has been used for centuries. This non-invasive diagnostic tool involves testing a large muscle to provide feedback on energy blockages, nutritional deficiencies, and food sensitivities. For example, the subject being tested is given a food object to hold in one hand. The practitioner then pushes down on the subject's opposite arm to test for muscular strength. If the subject is holding a nutritious food such as broccoli, the muscle will strengthen and the upward force against the practitioner's downward pressure will be strong. If the subject is holding a substance that drains the body such as white sugar or caffeine, the muscle will weaken.

When I first heard of this test, I was very skeptical. However, when comparing it against other diagnostics (such as the ELISA test), I found it surprisingly accurate in determining food allergies. The key to the success of this technique lies in the capability and expertise of the health care practitioner.

Vega and Interro Testing

Vega and Interro tests are not considered mainstream diagnostics and are used mostly by doctors practising environmental medicine and/or by naturopaths. A Vega test checks for changes in a person's skin conductivity following the application of a small voltage. Acupuncture points are used to check for electronic disturbances while the subject holds an electrode to maintain the flow of energy. Food sources are tested individually in homeopathic doses sealed in ampoules. It is thought that a negative electronic disturbance is an indication of a negative reaction to the food source. Interro testing is similar except instead of using food ampoules, a computerized program is used to detect food reactions. There has not been much research on the validity and reliability of these tests. In my practice, I have found them to be fairly accurate and useful in conjunction with other diagnostics. The cost of a Vega or Interro test is significantly cheaper than the ELISA test, ranging from approximately $85 to $110.

Pulse Test

The pulse test is a technique you can use at home to determine food allergies. Take your pulse with your index finger for one minute. A normal pulse rate is between fifty-two and seventy beats per minute. After taking your normal pulse rate, eat the food in question. If the suspected food is dairy, eat it by itself (that is, do not eat cheese on a slice of bread) to ensure that the allergy is to the dairy and not to the bread. Wait approximately fifteen to twenty minutes after eating the food and retake your pulse. If your pulse has sped up more than ten beats per minute, eliminate the food and retest yourself within a month.[2]

PREVENTING FOOD ALLERGIES NATURALLY

Can food allergies really be prevented? What if both parents are allergy sufferers? While it is true that having a genetic predisposition toward allergies definitely increases the odds of a child developing allergies, there are certain nutritional steps that can help to safeguard or lessen the severity of an allergic response. This is especially true for food allergies. In a child's first year of life, when the immune system is still developing, there is a small window of opportunity to establish a foundation of optimal intestinal health. Strong digestive health and proper nutrition and absorption are the best insurance policies to ward off the development of future food allergies and food sensitivities.

Breast Is Best!

Numerous studies have clearly identified breast milk as one of the most effective elements in protecting against the development of allergies. Children who are breast-fed tend to suffer less from allergies, asthma, digestive disorders, and eczema. A mother's milk passes on protective antibodies to a baby's delicate system, setting the stage for long-lasting immunity. Breast milk is filled with white blood cells and immunoglobins that are extremely efficient at warding off potential infections. Specifically, the immunoglobin IgA provides unparalleled protection for a baby's immature digestive system. A breast-fed baby's digestive system also contains large amounts of lactobacillus bifidus, the beneficial bacteria that can ward off the growth of harmful microorganisms. Breast milk is a dynamic fluid that constantly changes to meet an infant's nutritional and developmental needs. For example, morning milk is different from evening milk, and breast milk when a baby is one month old is different from breast milk when a baby is three months old. The protein, fat, and carbohydrate blend is continuously adapting to a baby's growing body. Breast milk provides a complete source of nutrition for babies until they are four to six months old, when solid foods are ready to be introduced.

For every breast-fed baby who gets chronic diarrhea, 100 bottle-fed babies have the same problem.

Some of my female patients stop breast-feeding, attributing their children's colic, crying, or constipation to a breast milk allergy. This is simply not true. *A child is never allergic to the mother's breast milk, only to something the mother is eating while nursing.* If a strictly breast-fed baby begins to show signs of an allergic response or colic, the mother's diet should be investigated. Often the problem is cow's milk in the form of cheese, yogurt, ice cream, or milk, which must be eliminated from the mother's diet. Cow's milk is significantly more protein dense than human milk, and can overtax a newborn's system. Casein is one of the proteins in cow's milk that appears to be responsible for most allergic responses. Signs to watch out for are a chronic runny nose, respiratory distress, vomiting or spitting up, poor digestion (colic, runny stool, or constipation), and skin rashes. A mother can perform an elimination diet on herself by removing suspected food culprits and monitoring her infant's reaction. Eliminating the suspected food for a month should be enough to identify the food trigger.

The most recent findings indicate that only about 20 percent of all infants are breast-fed until the age of five to six months.[3]

In addition to the advantages of breast milk, women also secrete a nutritionally dense fluid called colostrum, a thick, sticky fluid that is secreted for approximately three days before a mother's milk arrives. This vital liquid gold is full of nutritional benefits for a newborn. Colostrum acts as a laxative to jump-start an infant's digestive system, is loaded with protective antibodies, and contains essential amino acids for proper growth and development. Colostrum also seals off the permeable gaps in a baby's immature intestinal tract. If you are able to breast-feed but have decided not to, I encourage you to give your children the gift of colostrum. The immunity and protection a child receives from it in the first three days of life is immeasurable.

One year has been shown to be the optimal amount of time to breast-feed. If a year is not an option, a minimum of six weeks is thought to be best. A child's immune system is especially susceptible to infection in the first six weeks of life and is dependent on the protection received through mother's milk. For more information on breast-feeding or if you are having difficulty feeding your child, contact La Leche League in Canada at www.lalecheleague.org or at 1-800-665-4324 for personal consultations. In the United States, contact 847-519-7730 for referrals.

In addition to protection against allergies, breast-feeding has numerous other health benefits.

The pros of breast-feeding for an infant are:

- Contributes to mouth and jaw development
- Disease-preventing immunity is passed on to child
- Fewer incidence of diarrhea or colic
- Fewer respiratory and ear infections
- Higher IQs
- Reduced incidence of cancer
- Reduced incidence of sudden infant death syndrome (SIDS)
- Reduced occurrence of Type I diabetes
- Straighter teeth

The benefits for mothers are:

- Reduced risk of ovarian and breast cancer
- Bonding with child
- Easier weight loss

If nursing is not an option for you, if the baby is not latching, if you have had breast surgery, or if you are taking certain medications, etc., do not worry. There are other options that can help protect your infant against the development of future allergies. In truth, there is no formula available that can match the benefits of breast milk, so supplementation will be necessary. Doctors typically recommend either a dairy- or soy-based formula. If you choose a dairy-based formula, I recommend selecting one that has been hydrolyzed (protein hydrolysate or predigested formula will be on the label). This type of formula has been specially treated to break down milk protein into smaller, more absorbable protein units and has been shown to be less allergenic. Standard dairy formulas that have not been hydrolyzed put considerable stress on an immature digestive system, resulting in allergic reactions in infants. Research shows that a later introduction of cow's milk into your children's diet may delay the onset of allergies. According to Dr. Galland, MD, author of *Superimmunity for Kids*:

> *Cow's milk in the first year or too early feeding of solid food will precipitate allergies. Why? Because an infant's intestinal tract is porous; it can't screen out the big molecules that cause allergies. This is why infants under a year old are particularly susceptible to food allergies, and why you should not feed an infant wheat, cow's milk, fish, or egg whites during the first year of life. It takes six to twelve months for an infant's intestinal tract to develop the ability to screen out allergenic molecules.*[4]

Classic signs and symptoms of milk intolerance in newborns are skin reactions, spitting up, diarrhea, colic, chronic crying, and breathing problems. Sadly, I have seen far too many infants on puffers and steroids for respiratory infections that have cleared up when dairy was eliminated from their diet.

In one recent study from Arizona State University, researchers found that the early ingestion of cow's milk-based formulas significantly increased the risk of a child developing diabetes.

If a child has a reaction to a hydrolyzed dairy formula, try a non-genetically modified soy formula (non-GMO). Many kids who are allergic to dairy formulas might also show an allergic response to soy formulas. If this is the case, speak to your doctor about elemental formulas or goat's milk, which is currently not sold as a commercialized formula and should be used as a last resort. Goat's milk is also deficient in folic acid and vitamin B12, so supplementation will be necessary. If goat's milk is the only option left, speak to a naturopath, midwife, or birthing center familiar with making homemade goat's milk formula.

Formulas are an attempt to mimic nature and are therefore still deficient in certain nutrients. Most are deficient in omega-3 essential fatty acids. I highly recommend supplementing a formula-fed baby with an omega-3 supplement. Simply divide ½–1 teaspoon of fish oil or flaxseed oil into a bottle over the course of two or three feedings. Remember, these oils should never be heated and if a smell is detected, they should be discarded immediately.

Clean Out the Pipes

In an ideal state, the digestive system's job is to properly absorb, digest, and distribute nutrients throughout the bloodstream, thereby nourishing surrounding organs. In addition to these functions, the digestive system is also equipped with good bacteria whose job is to kill off any harmful microbes. Unfortunately, certain foods, medications, high stress levels, refined foods, and lack of fresh water make the digestive system's job extremely difficult. One of the sure signs of an overworked and weak digestive system is the development of allergies. When we clean up the intestinal tract, allergy symptoms lessen and even subside. I encourage parents of allergic children to pay attention to the state of their children's diet and digestive strength. It is not uncommon to have a child who suffers from irritable bowel syndrome, also develop a skin allergy such as eczema or, for a child who has had their healthy intestinal flora wiped out by repeated doses of antibiotics suffer from frequent ear or respiratory infections. For the best results, allergies must be addressed from the inside out.

The most common causes leading to a weak digestive system are:

- Metabolic stress and overload
- Overuse of antibiotics
- Poor diet
- Undersecretion of stomach acid and or pancreatic enzymes

The good bacterium in our digestive system is essential for the digestion of food. As mentioned earlier, antibiotics destroy the good and the bad bacteria in a child's digestive system, leaving room for the overgrowth of unhealthy microbes such as yeast, bacteria, and viruses. The body's immune system reacts to these microbes by forming an immune response called an antigen-antibody complex. Antigen-antibody complexes attack the lining of the intestinal tract, causing an inflammatory response, diarrhea, constipation, and cramping. In addition, these immune complexes can travel through the blood, creating a multitude of symptoms including inflammation in joints (arthritis), respiratory upset (asthma), and frequent infections (ear and throat). What is commonly diagnosed as an allergy may have been prompted by a deficiency of good bacteria. Without restoring a child's proper bowel flora with a probiotic such as acidophilus or bifidus supplementation, the allergic response is likely to recur. For breast-feeding mothers, bifidus powder should be put on the nipple to ensure it is absorbed into the baby's digestive system.

Another cause of allergies is leaky gut syndrome. Depending on where and how the body's immune system reacts, leaky gut syndrome can create allergic symptoms such as wheezing, fatigue, weight gain, mood swings, sneezing, and coughing. The goal is to heal the gut and to improve the allergic state with the following techniques:

- Remove all food allergies and sensitivities. If you are unsure which foods your children are allergic to, try following the elimination diet outlined above.

- Supplement with a probiotic (either acidophilus or bifidus, depending on your children's ages).

- Supplement with ½–1 teaspoon of fish oil or flaxseed oil daily.

- Remove acid-forming foods such as refined carbohydrates, sugars, meats, and dairy.

- Drink filtered water. Avoid sugary juices, pop, and other caffeinated beverages.

- Ensure your children are eating fresh vegetables, fruits, and whole grains.

- Supplement your children's diet with an extra dose of fruits and vegetables by adding a green powder such as greens+ kids into their daily regime.

When first introducing solid foods into a newborn's system, it is best to wait until the baby is four to six months old. Foods should be introduced one at a time, starting with mushy cereals such as oatmeal and pureed vegetables including broccoli, squash, kale, and yams. Proteins such as lean meats and chicken should not be introduced until the child is ten months old. As mentioned, dairy should not be introduced for at least a year.

Once a child is more than a year old, most foods are acceptable. Try to keep the anti-nutrient foods such as sugar, preservatives, fried foods, and food coloring to a minimum. Also, it is best to include a large variety of food choices in your children's diet. As you now know, the body does not like to receive the same foods over and over again.

Hydrochloric Acid Secretion

The last possible causes of an unhealthy digestive system are an insufficient amount of hydrochloric acid secreted by the stomach and/or a deficiency in protease, the enzyme secreted in the stomach to break down proteins. A deficiency in hydrochloric acid (a condition known as hypochlorydia) is actually more common than an overproduction of acid. In addition, hypochlorydia and improper enzyme secretion have been implicated as one of the potential causes of food allergies. As mentioned, food allergies and sensitivities are often triggered by undigested food particles or by large protein molecules. An enzyme supplement (available in chewable, capsule, or powder form) can assist in cleaning up the intestinal system, making digestion of food somewhat easier.

Top Supplements for Allergies in Children

In addition to diet, there are certain supplements that can help to ward off and even reverse an allergy state in a child. The following are the top picks that should be used if your child is an allergy sufferer:

- Fish oil or flaxseed oil to reduce inflammatory response
- Green powder that can be mixed into juice (greens+ kids)
- High-quality multivitamin
- Probiotic (acidophilus or bifidus, depending on age)
- Vitamin C (500–1,000 milligrams)

TRY

1. Including a wide variety of healthy selections in your children's diet to prevent food sensitivities. Your children's favorite foods are usually the ones they develop an intolerance to.

   ▪

2. Filling your children's diet with vitamin C and other bioflavonoids found in fruits and green and orange vegetables. These foods help to protect the body against allergens, boost immunity, and reduce the inflammatory response naturally.

   ▪

3. Eliminating anti-nutrient foods from your children's diet, such as white sugar, caffeine, food dyes, preservatives, and aspartame.

   ▪

4. Supplementing with fish oil or flaxseed oil (½–1 teaspoon) or a supplement that contains a high amount of DHA, (the absorbable derivative of flaxseed oil). Include foods that contain omega-3 essential fatty acids such as walnuts, seeds, salmon, tuna, and omega-3 eggs.

   ▪

5. Eliminating funny fats such as partially hydrogenated and hydrogenated oils. These contribute to the development and worsening of allergies.

NOTES

1 M. Murray and J. Pizzorno, *Encyclopaedia of Natural Medicine* (New York: Prima Health, 1998).

2 J. Balch and P. Balch, *Prescriptions for Nutritional Healing* (New York: Avery Publishing Group, 1997).

3 http://nutrition.about.com

4 L. Galland, *Superimmunity for Kids* (New York: Dell Publishing, 1988).

CHAPTER 11

Ear Infections

I T IS A TERRIBLE scene to watch. Your young children, who can't ver-
balize their discomfort, start tugging at their ears and whimpering
with pain. You quickly recognize this as the beginning of another full-
blown ear infection and rush to the doctor, who hands you a prescription. Although you are a bit concerned that your children have already
been on antibiotics twice that year for similar complaints, you fill the
prescription and hope for the best. Disaster averted or vicious cycle
perpetuated?

In North America, 25 million children annually will visit doctors for
the treatment of middle ear infections, otherwise called acute otitis media
(AOM). Middle ear infections are by far the most common pediatric
complaint. The prescribed treatment for ear infections is usually antibiotics. As mentioned in an earlier chapter the
indiscriminate use of antibiotics is creating a
resistance and the development of super bugs.
Science's attempt to kill bacteria permanently
in a child's system is not working. A more sen-
sible and effective approach is to investigate
the root cause of ear infections and to prevent
their development in the first place.

> *It has been estimated that as
> many as 95 percent of all chil-
> dren suffer from at least one ear
> infection by the age of six.*[1]

WHAT IS AOM?

Acute otitis media is caused by inflammation of the inner ear. The middle ear is connected to the nasal cavity and the throat by the Eustachian
tube. A blockage of the Eustachian tubes can occur because of a cold,

allergy, or upper respiratory infection, which can then lead to a buildup of fluid behind the eardrum. Children under the age of six are more likely than older children to develop middle ear infections because their Eustachian tubes are more horizontal than an adult's, making drainage of fluids more difficult. If fluid builds up in the middle ear, an infection can result. The typical symptoms of AOM in a child are:

- Crying and irritability
- Difficulty hearing
- Ear drainage
- Fever
- Pain
- Pulling on the ear

Ear infections should not to be taken lightly. For starters, they are the most common cause of hearing loss in a child. Also, because of their close proximity to other important structures in the head such as the mastoid bone, it is important to ensure that the infection does not spread. As mentioned earlier, in conventional medicine, antibiotics such as amoxicillin are typically chosen as the first line of defense. Unfortunately, this method of treatment may not be as effective as once thought. Current research shows that antibiotics may be necessary in acute situations; however, their repetitive use does not appear to lessen the recurrence of future ear infections. In fact, studies show that the indiscriminate use of antibiotics may even increase the development of future ear infections in a child. Consider the following facts on the use of antibiotics and ear infections:

- Six out of seven children do not respond to antibiotic therapy.

- Further attacks are just as likely to happen even after antibiotics.

- There is no evidence that using an antibiotic makes a child less likely to be deaf one month to three months after an infection.

- The unnecessary use of antibiotics can increase the risk of super bugs, which can resist antibiotics in the future should more serious illnesses develop in your children.[2]

In contrast to the North American medical approach to ear infections, other countries such as the Netherlands have a wait-and-see approach to AOM. In the Netherlands, children over the age of two with ear infections are monitored for one or two days to see if their condition improves. In one study it was found that over 80 percent of children with AOM recovered from the pain and fever of an uncomplicated ear infection within twenty-four hours of a diagnosis without an antibiotic. The rate of bacterial resistance in the Netherlands is about 1 percent compared to approximately 25 percent in the United States.[3]

If antibiotics repeatedly fail, the next step typically taken is a procedure called a myringotomy and a tympanostomy, otherwise known as draining and putting tubes in a child's ears. This procedure is performed under general anesthetic, and a surgeon inserts tiny plastic tubes into a child's middle ear to promote drainage of fluid. The effectiveness and side effects of tympanostomies are controversial. The surgery involves puncturing a hole in your child's eardrum and inserting a tube. This can result in loss of hearing from scarring or hardening of the eardrum. Eventually when the hole in the eardrum closes, the tube can fall out, requiring further surgical interventions.

CAUSES OF AOM?

There are various causes that can predispose a child to developing AOM. Research shows that the most common causes are:

- Food allergies
- Formula-feeding instead of breast-feeding
- Second-hand smoke
- Bottle drinking while lying on back

Food Allergies and Sensitivities

When a child arrives in my office with recurring ear infections, my first question to the parent is always, "Does your child consume dairy products?" Often chronic ear infections can be stopped by removing all dairy products from the diet. The consumption of dairy products increases mucous production, allowing an environment for harmful bacteria and viruses to proliferate. In addition to excess mucous production, dairy products can cause an inflammation in the ear canal that can trigger or worsen a pre-existing condition. I recommend eliminating all dairy products (which includes milk, cheese, yogurt, and ice cream) for a six to eight week period and substituting with tasty soy or rice products. Some soy and rice imitation products are delicious and some are not. If your children do not like the first one you purchase, try another product. Refer to Appendix I for some delicious dairy-free alternatives available at most health food stores and some grocery stores. If your children are still bottle-feeding and suffering from ear infections, try switching to a soy or rice formula. In addition to removing dairy, it is best to boost their immunity with the supplements outlined in the section below.

If the removal of dairy does not eliminate the ear infections, other common food allergies should be investigated and removed one by one from your children's diet. Anti-nutrient foods can also weaken the immune system, leaving children more predisposed to ear infections. Remove all anti-nutrient foods from their diet to help keep the immune system strong and healthy.

RECOMMENDED SUPPLEMENTS FOR EAR INFECTIONS

These top supplements will reduce inflammation in the inner ear, restore good bacteria, and boost immunity to ward off future ear infections. They are available in kid-friendly forms such as powders, chewable tablets, and have natural flavoring. Visit your local health food store to see the varieties they carry.

Remember, supplements do not replace a healthy diet. It is important to use supplements in conjunction with and not as a replacement for healthy eating and exercise.

Acidophilus

It is important to get the good bacteria back into children's systems to help them fight off infections. This is especially true for children who have been on several courses of antibiotics. A supplement of the probiotic acidophilus in capsule or powdered form in your children's juice, applesauce, or food will replenish their microflora to a balanced, healthy state. Probiotics should be used as a supplement following a course of antibiotics, not at the same time.

Fish or Flaxseed Oil

Fish oils and flaxseed oil contain omega-3 essential fatty acids that reduce the inflammation caused by acute otitis media. Once inflammation has been reduced, pain will also begin to subside. Adding fish oil or flaxseed oil to juice, applesauce, or salad dressings will give your children more of the fats essential for optimal health. I recommend supplementing with ½–1 teaspoon of fish or flaxseed oil daily or 2 teaspoons in divided doses for infections. For an added omega-3 boost for the entire family, try making the following delicious flaxseed oil salad dressing.

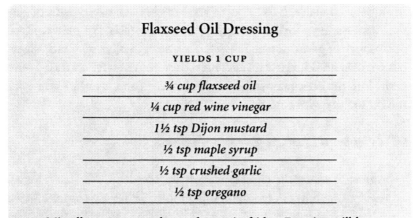

Flaxseed Oil Dressing

YIELDS 1 CUP

¾ cup flaxseed oil
¼ cup red wine vinegar
1½ tsp Dijon mustard
½ tsp maple syrup
½ tsp crushed garlic
½ tsp oregano

Mix all contents together and store in fridge. Dressing will last five to seven days.

Vitamin C and a Mixture of Bioflavonoids

Vitamin C is one of the most effective vitamins for boosting immunity and battling infections. It also contains antihistamine properties that can be beneficial if ear infections are due to an allergic response. A child can be supplemented with 500–1,000 milligrams of vitamin C per day. For children, chewable vitamin C tablets are recommended. If they experience diarrhea, cut back on the dosage. In addition to a supplement, be sure to include foods that are rich in vitamin C such as fresh berries, citrus fruits, and broccoli.

Zinc

Zinc is essential for the proper functioning of the immune system and helps to battle infections. Most children and adults are somewhat deficient in zinc because of our depleted soil. Children can suck on zinc lozenges while suffering from an ear or respiratory infection. Zinc lozenges are available at most health food stores.

Garlic

Garlic is one of the most potent natural antibiotics and immune system stimulators available. If a child is old enough to swallow a capsule of garlic, purchase the odorless form to avoid any protests. For pain control, boil a clove of garlic in water, mash and add it to olive oil. Once the oil has cooled and is lukewarm, add a few drops of the olive oil mixed with garlic into the ear canal while the child is lying on his or her side. Pack the ear loosely with cotton.

Other Natural Choices for Ear Infections

- **Water:** Ensure your child is well hydrated with fresh water, herbal teas, broths, and diluted natural fruit juices. Eliminate sugary juices.

- **Chiropractic care:** A chiropractor is trained to determine if spinal motion is normal. When spinal motion is restricted in a child's upper neck area, otherwise called the cervical spine, nerve interference can make an ear infection more likely to occur.

- **Massage therapy:** Pediatric massage therapy encourages lymphatic drainage, enabling potential viruses and/or bacteria to drain from the ear canal.

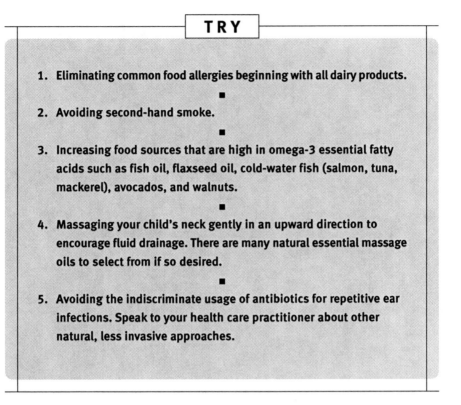

TRY

1. Eliminating common food allergies beginning with all dairy products.

   ■

2. Avoiding second-hand smoke.

   ■

3. Increasing food sources that are high in omega-3 essential fatty acids such as fish oil, flaxseed oil, cold-water fish (salmon, tuna, mackerel), avocados, and walnuts.

   ■

4. Massaging your child's neck gently in an upward direction to encourage fluid drainage. There are many natural essential massage oils to select from if so desired.

   ■

5. Avoiding the indiscriminate usage of antibiotics for repetitive ear infections. Speak to your health care practitioner about other natural, less invasive approaches.

NOTES

1 J. Balch and P. Balch, *Prescriptions for Nutritional Healing* (New York: Avery Publishing Group, 1997).

2 http://www.medinfo.co.uk/conditions/otitism-antib.html

3 http://www.chiropracticresearch.org

CHAPTER 12

Ulcerative Colitis, Crohn's, and Irritable Bowel Syndrome

I N THE PAST few decades, digestive disorders such as Crohn's disease, ulcerative colitis, and irritable bowel syndrome have increased dramatically. Unfortunately, more children and teenagers now suffer from these digestive disorders than ever before. Several youngsters ranging from six to eighteen have come to my office, suffering from very severe intestinal symptoms. Gastrointestinal illness can take its toll at any age, but it is especially difficult for children. Along with the proper tools for healing and nourishment, these children and young adults need a significant amount of emotional support from parents and caretakers. Not only are they afraid of eating because of pain, uncontrolled bowel movements, and/or severe cramping, they also feel isolated and quite different from other children. As mentioned earlier, children do not like to feel different from their peers. It is important to address children's concerns as stress can worsen all bowel conditions. Reassure them that every step will be taken to help heal their bowels, thereby restoring them to a normal lifestyle. If your children are in school, it is wise to alert school personnel about their illness. Explain any special dietary needs and ways that teachers can help them to cope.

In this chapter, I will divide digestive disorders into two categories:

1. Inflammatory bowel diseases: Crohn's disease and ulcerative colitis
2. Non-inflammatory bowel diseases: irritable bowel syndrome

INFLAMMATORY BOWEL DISEASES IN CHILDREN

Crohn's disease and ulcerative colitis are both classified as inflammatory bowel diseases that often mimic each other in presenting symptoms. The main difference lies in the area of the intestinal tract affected. Crohn's disease affects the entire lining of the intestinal wall and can occur anywhere from the mouth to the anus. Ulcerative colitis involves only two layers of the intestinal wall, the mucosa and submucosa, and typically occurs in the colon.

Malabsorption syndrome and malnutrition are of great concern in children suffering from these conditions. Ensuring that growing children receive adequate caloric intake is of the utmost importance. In addition, if intestinal bleeding is occurring (blood in the child's stool), anemia may result and also must be addressed.

Before introducing proper nutrition, the injured area of the digestive tract must be healed. Covering up the injured part of the intestinal tract with medications or merely introducing healthier foods will not work over the long term. The underlying problem must be addressed first.

In the United States, it is estimated that 1 million people suffer from Crohn's or colitis. Ten percent, or an estimated 100,000, of those afflicted are under eighteen.

An injured intestinal wall can be compared to a skinned knee. If the knee is continually irritated and a scab is not given the opportunity to form and protect the underlying injury, the knee does not have the chance to heal properly. The same is true for the intestinal wall. If the intestinal tract is continually irritated by foods such as refined sugars and dairy, stress, lack of water, and poor bowel flora due to antibiotics, it will not heal. If healing does not take place first, proper absorption, digestion, and excretion cannot occur. There are many situations in which the intestinal wall has become so inflamed and injured that medication such as corticosteroids are necessary to halt inflammation and prevent a bowel obstruction. Natural health changes such as those outlined below in "Dr. Joey's Intestinal Healing Protocol" can be made while a child is on medication.

Inflammatory bowel diseases (IBD) occur most often between the ages of fifteen to thirty-five, but are now being diagnosed in younger populations. Females are affected slightly more than males, and people of Jewish background have an incidence that is three to six times higher compared with people of non-Jewish heritage.[1] IBD are most common in developed countries (Canada, the United States, and Europe), and are more prevalent in urban than rural regions.

Crohn's Disease

Crohn's disease can occur anywhere along the intestinal tract; however, it usually is found in the small intestine. The disease is characterized by chronic and long-lasting areas of inflammation that can result in scar formation and narrowing of the tract. Because the primary role of the intestinal tract is for nutrient absorption, children suffering from Crohn's disease often have several vitamin and mineral deficiencies. Symptoms of Crohn's disease are:

- Bleeding (red or black stools)
- Cramping
- Delayed growth and sexual maturation
- Fever
- Frequent diarrhea
- Headache
- Joint pain
- Lack of energy
- Loss of appetite
- Nausea
- Pain in upper and/or lower quadrant
- Steatorrhea (the presence of excess fat in the stool)
- Weight loss

People suffering from Crohn's disease normally have flare-ups or attacks, which may occur every few months or once or twice a year.

Ulcerative Colitis

As mentioned, ulcerative colitis shares many common features with Crohn's disease.

Ulcerative colitis (UC) typically occurs in the lower bowel and colon, specifically the lower left section of the large intestine called the sigmoid colon—see page 47 for diagram. The disease is characterized by ulcer development in the mucous membranes of the intestinal wall. The colon is responsible for stool compaction and proper elimination. Because of the ulcer formation, the injured colon muscles are overworked and can develop small pouch-like projections called diverticula. Signs and symptoms of ulcerative colitis are:

- Delayed growth and sexual maturation
- Fever and fatigue
- Frequent diarrhea with blood (can occur several times daily)
- Gas and bloating
- Joint pain
- Lack of energy
- Occasional hard stools
- Pain
- Weight loss

The most accurate diagnostic test available to differentiate between Crohn's and UC is an endoscopic exam in which a flexible tube is inserted into the rectum to allow doctors to view the internal lining of the digestive organs. The inflammation of ulcerative colitis will tend to show in uniform, continuous areas, whereas in Crohn's disease inflamed areas of intestine tend to alternate with healthy sections. Often preparation for this test is more stressful than the test itself. Fasting or drinking clear fluids, laxatives, and enemas may be necessary to clear the bowel before the test. Children anxious about this procedure are sometimes sedated to make the experience less traumatic.

> *Children and teenagers who suffer from Crohn's or colitis are at greater risk of developing colon cancer.*

Causes of Inflammatory Bowel Diseases

The underlying causes of Crohn's and colitis are unknown. Theories about the causes of IBD include the following:

- Antibiotic exposure
- Autoimmune disease

- Diet containing fast foods, refined foods, sugar, and a deficiency of fiber
- Food allergies
- Genetic predisposition
- Overgrowth of candida (yeast)
- Parasitic infection

As mentioned, stress can definitely worsen children's digestive disorders. Whether it is school, friends, home life, or the disorder itself, it is best to sit down with a child to talk about how you can help them deal with their anxiety.

Important Question for Parents to Consider

The following questions can help to determine underlying conditions that may trigger IBD. Do you answer yes to any of the following?

1. Have your children been on antibiotics in the past year?

2. Were they on antibiotics frequently as infants or toddlers?

3. Were they bottle fed instead of breast-fed?

4. Were they colicky as babies?

5. Did they ever suffer from thrush (an overgrowth of candida albicans or yeast in the mouth)?

6. Do they have food cravings?

7. Do they consume dairy? Fast foods? Refined carbohydrates?

These questions can help you find the underlying cause of IBD.

Conventional Treatment for Inflammatory Bowel Disease

Currently, there are two standard approaches for treating inflammatory bowel disease: medication and surgery. The medications used to treat IBD decrease inflammation in the intestinal tract. In moderate to severe cases of IBD, corticosteroids (the most popular being prednisone) are used as a first line of defence. Although prednisone is effective and necessary in certain cases, it does not address underlying problems (healing the injured area of the bowel). In addition, the side effects of this drug can be quite severe, including weight gain, acne, facial hair, hypertension, mood swings, and increased risk of infection. It can also cause "prednisone moonface" meaning a child's face will puff out and swell. This effect can have negative social and psychological effects for children who are trying to fit in and want to look like their other friends. One of the most serious consequences of long-term corticosteroid use is the loss of calcium from the bone matrix. Patients who are on prednisone for long periods are encouraged to have frequent bone density tests to ensure that they have not developed osteopenia (significant bone loss). Many researchers have suggested that prolonged corticosteroid use (more than one year) is one of the major causes of reduced bone density.

If medications do not prove effective in the treatment of IBD, surgery is often the next step. Surgery is typically considered if there is massive bleeding, a blockage, or if side effects of the medication have become too severe. Depending on the location of the injured area in the intestinal tract, patients will undergo a bowel resection and have the unhealthy area of their digestive system, whether small or large intestine, removed. One of the most common surgeries for colitis patients is called an ileostomy. This procedure involves removing the colon and the rectum and attaching a pouch to the terminal ileum for excretion. The pouch, worn over the opening to collect waste, needs to be emptied by the patient. This situation is obviously far from ideal for children and teenagers.

Illnesses That May Accompany IBD

IBD begins in the intestinal system, but may affect many other parts of the body such as the joints, skin, eyes, and liver. As mentioned, it is speculated that IBD and related illnesses may be an autoimmune response. An autoimmune reaction occurs when the body launches an attack (called an antigen-antibody response) against its own tissues or organs. Examples of these extraintestinal manifestations are:

- Anemia
- Arthritis
- Dry eyes

- Eczema
- Gallstones
- Irregular menstruation
- Kidney stones
- Liver disease (fatty liver, cirrhosis, chronic active hepatitis)
- Uveits (inflammation of the middle layer of the eye wall that may cause sensitivity to light, blurred vision, pain, and redness)
- Weakness and fatigue

Twenty-five percent of people diagnosed with IBD will suffer from arthritis.

Dr. Joey's Intestinal Healing Protocol

Depending on the severity and progression of your children's IBD, healing will be different from child to child. I have seen children suffering from the worst cases of IBD respond to

The Herxheimer response is a medical term that refers to problems generated by a detoxification process (healing of the intestinal system). This response can result in flu-like symptoms.

dietary and supplement therapies. However, every case is different and there are certain cases where the progression of the disease is too advanced to respond. It is always best to consult your doctor when planning to make dietary changes. Healing can take anywhere from four to twelve weeks before an improvement is noticed. It is also not uncommon in the first month for children to feel worse before they feel better. While the digestive system is being cleaned up from the inside out, the body rids itself of toxins that can worsen symptoms before they subside. The most common symptoms experienced in the first month are fatigue, white coating over the tongue, weight loss, constipation, headaches, diarrhea, and acne. This effect is called the Herxheimer response.

The Goals

Parents often ask me how they will know when their children's intestinal tract has begun to heal. The best indicator is the cessation of symptoms. For example, within four to twelve weeks, parents should begin to notice some of the following taking place:

- Ability to digest raw fruits and vegetables without cramping or other abdominal responses
- Brighter, less dry eyes

- Cessation of skin conditions
- Decrease or cessation of pain in joints
- Increase in energy
- Normal bowel movements (once a day without strain, mucous, or blood)
- Rosy color returning to cheeks

You may also consider asking your doctor about having a follow-up colonoscopy or ultrasound done within three to six months to note changes that have taken place.

Fifteen Food Rules for Intestinal Health

I recommend the following 15 food rules for children suffering from active IBD. By active IBD, I mean frequent bouts of diarrhea, blood in stool, pain, and cramping. The dietary changes outlined below can be followed with or without medication. Although these dietary changes may feel slightly restrictive at first, it is necessary to follow them as much as possible to give the intestinal tract the proper environment to heal. Please refer to Appendix I for delicious, dairy-free, wheat-free products.

1. Eliminate all processed and refined foods such as white sugar and white refined floury products.

2. Eliminate potential food allergens. Dairy is the most common food allergen. Without its complete elimination, healing is compromised. The only exception is a yogurt-like product called kefir. Kefir is available in most health food stores, is very alkalizing, and helps to soothe the intestinal wall.

3. Substitute dairy products with rice or soy versions of cheese slices, cream cheese, Parmesan cheese, and ice cream. Try to alternate between soy and rice products. Children who suffer from IBD can also be sensitive to soy. If this is the case, use only rice products. When purchasing these food items, try to find those that do not contain casein in the ingredients.

4. Substitute wheat products with brown rice breads, pastas, or rice. When cooking brown rice pasta or rice, overcook for the first four to six weeks to make it mushy and easy to absorb. Other grains that may be tolerated are millet, buckwheat, kamut, or spelt.

5. Avoid eating toast or barbequed foods for the first six weeks.

6. No nuts, seeds, raisins, or popcorn.

7. All vegetables should be eaten overcooked or pureed. Raw vegetables are wrapped in cellulose and can be very difficult to digest for a compromised digestive system. If the IBD is very severe, organic, pureed vegetable baby food is an option that should be considered.

8. Avoid mushrooms and melons—they promote the growth of fungus.

9. The only fruits that should be eaten in the first four to six weeks are mushy bananas, baked apples, or natural fruit juices. All berries should be avoided because of the seeds.

10. Include alkalizing juices such as natural or fresh-squeezed carrot, apple, grape, and pineapple juice.

11. Eliminate all red meats. Substitute with cold-water fish (salmon, tuna, mackerel three to five times per week). Omega-3 eggs and occasional chicken are acceptable options. Veggie burgers are also a great alternative for kids. (In severe cases of IBD, children are not able to break down the protein molecules of fish, chicken, or eggs. If this is the case, purchase liquid amino acids from your local health food store. Liquid amino acids are broken-down proteins that will ensure your children receive the building blocks necessary to heal and protect their developing bodies.)

12. Eliminate all trans-fatty acids, partially hydrogenated, or hydrogenated vegetable oils. These fats are commonly found in margarine, potato chips, salad dressings, and other processed and packaged baked goods. Olive oil should be used for cooking and flaxseed oil should be used for salad dressing.

13. Six to eight glasses of bottled water should be consumed daily. This helps to lessen the severity of a Herxheimer response.

14. Avoid all caffeine or carbonated beverages. Mint herbal tea is very healing and helpful for digestion.

15. Eliminate spices and spicy foods.

Once your children start to respond positively to this diet and show no symptoms for four weeks, other foods can *slowly* be reintroduced.

Raw, gaseous vegetables (lettuce, broccoli, spinach) should be one of the last food groups to try as they are very difficult to digest. Refer to Appendix IV for Dr. Joey's Supplements for healing UC and Crohn's

IRRITABLE BOWEL SYNDROME (IBS)

Irritable bowel syndrome is the most common intestinal disorder diagnosed in North America. It typically begins in adolescence, but is now being diagnosed in children as young as six. IBS does not fall under the category of inflammatory bowel diseases like Crohn's and colitis, and will therefore be dealt with separately. Unlike Crohn's and colitis, there are no physical findings for IBS and its root cause is not well understood. IBS is classified as a functional bowel disorder because it is caused by a problem in the mechanics of the bowel. The syndrome occurs with changes in the number and strength of contractions of the intestinal tract through which food passes. When the waves are fast and strong, diarrhea can occur. When the waves are slow, constipation typically follows.[2]

It is possible that IBS, which has no physical findings, can eventually lead to more serious conditions such as Crohn's or colitis that do have physical findings. Because IBS can often mimic other diseases or infections such as appendicitis, diverticulitis, Crohn's, or colitis, diagnosis should be made by a professional.

As mentioned, causes of IBS are unknown, but it may be related to:

- Diet consisting of processed foods
- Food sensitivities/allergies
- Parasite or candida (yeast) infection
- Stress

A stool sample taken by your doctor can indicate the presence of a parasite. Consider having this test done if your children are suffering from gastrointestinal complaints and have recently been to Mexico.

Symptoms of irritable bowel syndrome include:

- Bloating
- Constipation and/or diarrhea (often alternating)
- Gas

- Headaches
- Nausea
- Pain triggered by eating and relieved by a bowel movement

Dietary Approach to IBS

Unlike Crohn's and colitis in which fiber from raw fruits, vegetables, and grains can initially irritate the intestinal wall, fiber is recommended for the treatment of irritable bowel syndrome. The following foods can help alleviate IBS:

- Increase fruits, vegetables, and whole grains. Avoid using wheat bran as the choice of fiber. Many IBS kids are food sensitive, and wheat is one of the top allergens. Try using apples, oatbran, and legumes. Oatbran can be purchased in bulk from the health food store and can be added to your children's juice or used in baking.

- Eliminate possible food allergies such as dairy and wheat.

- Eliminate all processed foods and "funny fats" (fried foods, junk foods, chips, margarine, fast foods, etc.).

- Drink six to eight glasses of fresh distilled water daily. If necessary, add one quarter of fresh natural juice to your children's water to get them to drink it.

- If an intestinal upset occurs, switch to a bland, mushy diet. All fruits and vegetables should be cooked or pureed.

Supplements for IBS

- **Acidophilus:** ½ teaspoon/day or 2-3 capsules daily
- **Essential fatty acids:** One teaspoon of fish oil or flaxseed oil daily
- **Chewable digestive enzymes:** When necessary, if bloating occurs
- **Peppermint tea:** 1–2 lukewarm cups daily aids in digestion.

TRY

1. Having fresh, clean water available at all times.

    ■

2. Having your children discuss their concerns openly and assure them that every step will be taken to make them feel better.

    ■

3. Helping your children deal with their anxiety with methods such as belly breathing, positive visualization, and open conversation. Some children tend to "hold it in," and avoid going to the washroom when they need to. Depending on your children's ages, encourage them to pay attention to these signals by going to the bathroom when they feel the urge. Refer to the following chapter on stress busters for kids.

    ■

4. Eliminating all refined flours and possible food sensitivities. Remember, bread and pastas are not the enemy. The problem is in the refinement of flours and the wheat protein gluten. If a child is sensitive to wheat, there are many delicious pastas and breads made from healthier grains such as rice, millet or rye.

    ■

5. Supplementing with acidophilus, fish or flaxseed oils, and green powders.

NOTES

1 M. Murray and J. Pizzorno, *Encyclopaedia of Natural Medicine* (New York: Prima Health, 1998).

2 S. Gursche, *Encyclopedia of Natural Healing* (Burnaby, BC: alive books, 1997).

More Kid Factors for Optimal Health

Teach your children well.
—CROSBY, STILLS, NASH & YOUNG

By now you have discovered how essential an optimal diet filled with fresh, live, whole food is to the development of health and wellness in children. Although diet is the major ingredient in the recipe of health, there are other ingredients that also deserve our attention and consideration. Part IV addresses topics that are often overlooked in children, including natural sleep techniques, stress management, and the importance of drinking fresh, clean water. Answers to commonly asked questions about multivitamins, fevers, needs of the athletic child, etc., will also be provided in the final part of this section.

CHAPTER 13

MegaHealth for Kids

T HE BODY IS comprised of about 70 percent water. Next to air, water is the most vital substance the body needs to function properly. Water is involved in every aspect of your body's functions including digestion, excretion, and absorption of vital nutrients. It is responsible for maintaining normal body temperature, maintaining an acid/alkali environment in your system, and carrying out waste material from the body. You can survive for five weeks without food, but only five days without water.

YOU'RE NOT SICK, YOU'RE THIRSTY!

If after reading this book, you are contemplating which health change to implement first into your children's daily regime, pick water. Including fresh, clean water in your children's daily diet can relieve fatigue, asthma, allergies, arthritis, Crohn's, colitis, irritable bowel syndrome, and also assist with weight loss.

By the time children are thirsty, their bodies are already dehydrated. Unfortunately, many of them have switched to sugary pop and juice as replacements for water. In fact, children often report not feeling thirsty or losing the urge to drink. In an attempt to adapt to dehydration, children's bodies will eventually stop sending out signals of thirst, leaving them disconnected from their need for hydration. The good news is that after a few weeks of increasing children's daily water intake, their thirst will be reawakened. At this point, drinking water will not feel like a chore but an essential part of their daily routine.

So, how much water do children require on a daily basis? It depends on a child's age. Anywhere from six to eight glasses (each glass being 8 ounces) is recommended. In order to add more water to their diet, try watering down some natural juice. Send them to school with small bottles of water and consider investing in a water dispenser for the entire family. I guarantee you that if water is freely accessible in your kitchen, you and your children will start drinking more without even noticing it. Also, give them bottles of water when they engage in exercises such as bike riding or other sports so they can rehydrate properly.

> Beverages such as alcohol, coffee, soft drinks, and tea dehydrate the body. For every cup of coffee or soda drink consumed, replenish your children's systems with two glasses of water.

To avoid harmful microbes (such as E. coli and coliform), lead, copper, excess chlorine consumption, and many other toxins, I do not recommend drinking tap water. Children are even more susceptible than adults to these impurities. Alternatives such as steam, distilled, or reverse osmosis water are excellent choices.

SLEEP

The human body can survive only a limited amount of time without sleep. Most children between the ages of five and twelve sleep about eight to ten hours a night, although some need more than others. A normal sleep cycle consists of five stages. Stages 1 to 3 are considered light sleep, stage 4 is the deepest sleep, and stage 5 is known as rapid eye movement (REM) sleep. REM sleep occurs when children experience dreams that they may or may not remember. Children normally repeat stages 2, 3, 4, and REM about every ninety minutes, which is approximately four or five times a night.

How do you know if your children are getting enough sleep? Five to ten minutes after waking in the morning, they should rise feeling rested and ready to start their day. Once they are past the napping stage, a sufficient amount of sleep and proper rotation of the five sleep cycles should ensure they have enough energy and pep in their step to last the entire day. Irritability, falling asleep at school or in the car, and lack of motivation to participate in outdoor play or exercise may also be a sign of sleeping disorders. Sleeping patterns can also be affected by the timing of meals, food allergies, and the quality and quantity of food eaten.

Natural Tips for Kids to Catch Their zzzzzz's

- Try to get your children to go to bed at the same time every night—this helps them get into a sleep routine.

- Eliminate stimulant beverages at dinner or before bed. This includes sodas with caffeine and hot chocolate.

- Avoid watching television directly before bed. Scary movies or TV shows close to bedtime can make it difficult for children to fall asleep.

- Exercise is terrific for helping children sleep properly. However, do not let them exercise right before going to bed. Vigorous exercise in the evening will promote wakefulness.

- Depending on their ages, create a bedtime ritual for your children. This may include a bath, reading a book, discussing their day, or brushing their teeth. The key to a successful bedtime ritual is to create it and stick to it!

- Use lavender oil on their pillows or sheets. Lavender is a soft fragrance that calms and relaxes. Simply put a few drops on their bedding twenty minutes before bedtime. Keep the oil out of reach of children.

- Try using calming cassettes or music.

- Although eating a big meal prior to bedtime can inhibit sleep, certain foods in small doses can be very beneficial in sending them off to sleep. Bananas, figs, dates, yogurt, milk, tuna, turkey, and whole grain foods are high in tryptophan, which helps to promote sleep.

STRESS BUSTERS FOR KIDS

Similar to adults, children can feel stress and anxiety that can take a toll on their health. Without the skills or knowledge to express what they are feeling, stressed-out children can bottle up their emotions, creating negative effects both emotionally and physically. According to Dr. Hyla Cass, president of The Healthy Foundation and renowned psychiatrist, "during highly stressful times like these [in reference to post-September 11], children's bodies quickly use up their water-soluble vitamins such as Vitamin C, the B vitamins and folic acid. When these vitamins are depleted, it is more difficult for children to cope with their emotions."[1]

You know your children best. Some kids are more resilient than others to teasing, school issues, family situations, etc. I call these kids water-off-a-duck's-back children—nothing seems to bother them. Other children are more sensitive and require a little more attention, love, and affection. Try and meet your children's emotional needs by talking openly and paying attention to what may be bothering them. It is very hard to predict what will stress out a child and what will not. What may seem like a minor event to an adult, such as not being invited to a party, may seem catastrophic to a child. Practising stress management techniques with your children at an early age will open up the lines of communication with them and encourage them to share their problems. You will also feel reassured knowing that they will turn to you in times of stress.

Regardless of their ages, give your children special time with you. Often children need to feel they are safe and will be listened to before they will open up. When spending time with your children, don't pick up the phone or read e-mails, clean the kitchen or do a load of laundry. Devote that time to them. All the chores and phone calls will be there later, but the opportunity for a child to open up can easily pass. When your children have your complete attention, they will be more likely to confide in you. Here are some tips to help your kids reduce stress:

- Encourage your children to have a creative outlet for their emotions. Arts and crafts such as painting, drawing, and modeling clay can help them express their feelings and let off a little steam.

- Encourage your kids to exercise. There is nothing like a little sweat to take children's minds off their problems.

- Teach them the ancient art of yoga to develop coping skills. Home videos especially designed for kids are now available.

- Teach your children (and yourself!) how to belly breathe. During stressful situations, most of us breathe shallowly, not allowing a sufficient amount of oxygen into our lungs. Belly breathing involves taking deep breaths in through your nose for a count of five while your belly rises. Then exhale through your nose for a count of five while your stomach flattens. Children who are experiencing stress or a "fight or flight" response will become calmer by practising belly breathing several times a day.

- If they are old enough, encourage them to keep a journal or diary to record their feelings. Often writing things down on paper helps to ease stress.

- Bring laughter into your home. Rent funny movies, play board games, or tell jokes. Never underestimate the healing potential of laughter.

- Give them hugs, hugs, and more hugs. Children want to know that they will always be loved and supported.

COMMONLY ASKED QUESTIONS

In my practice, I have found there are certain repeating health topics that parents want more information on. The following are the answers to the questions I am most commonly asked.

Should My Children Take a Multivitamin?

Yes. Although I recommend that children should acquire most of their vitamins and minerals from whole foods, the reality is that it is quite difficult with today's processed foods. A high-quality daily powdered, chewable or liquid multivitamin can be just the sort of nutritional safety net they need. Research shows that providing vitamin supplements to at-risk children improves academic performance, decreases aggressive and violent behavior, and provides relief from stress and trauma.

It is best to introduce a multivitamin by a child's first birthday. Before that, children receive a sufficient amount of vitamins through breast milk or infant formula. Breast-fed babies may be prescribed a vitamin D supplement if they do not receive enough sun exposure. Your children's multivitamin should be taken with food in order to absorb the fat-soluble vitamins A, D, E, and K.

How Long Do Nutritional Changes Take to Make a Difference?

Nutritional changes vary from child to child. Because children do not have as much emotional or physical baggage as adults, they often respond faster. On average, parents typically notice a difference within three to six weeks of implementing nutritional changes. Remember, all kids, whether they are healthy or not, need a little nutritional fine-tuning. Even if the changes in your children's health are not overtly apparent, the underlying changes are enormous. Feel good about the quality of food you are providing for your family, knowing that it is promoting optimal health for your children. The focus is prevention, not treatment.

Should I Tell My Doctor About the Nutritional Changes I Am Making?

Of course! Food is the most powerful healing tool on the planet. I often have patients who hesitate to tell their doctor of the natural food changes they have made in their children's diet. Why not inform your doctor of these changes and allow him or her the opportunity to see the preventative and healing effects of foods? As doctors are just beginning to become informed in the area of nutrition, your testimonials and positive changes will only enhance your doctor's understanding. We are all in this game of health together. If your doctor does not support your dietary changes, that is okay. Making informed choices that you feel comfortable with is the most important thing.

How Can I Get My Children to Eat More Vegetables?

Dips, dips, and more dips! If your children resist eating the three to five servings of vegetables recommended daily, why not jazz them up a little with some tasty dips? My young nephews love guacamole, hummus (chickpea spread), or ranch dressing (dairy-free is available in health food stores).

Keep cut-up vegetables such as broccoli, carrots, snap peas, and cucumbers in Tupperware containers in the fridge for easily available snacks. When your child watches their favorite TV program, make sure they are munching on these whole, live foods rather than funny fat potato chips.

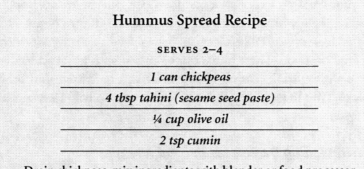

Hummus Spread Recipe

SERVES 2–4

1 can chickpeas

4 tbsp tahini (sesame seed paste)

¼ cup olive oil

2 tsp cumin

Drain chickpeas, mix ingredients with blender or food processor and enjoy!

Sweet Potato French Fries

SERVES 4–6

6 medium size sweet potatoes (yams)

¼ cup of extra virgin olive oil

2 tsp of seasoned salt

pepper to taste

Peel and cut sweet potatoes in ½-inch strips. With a pastry brush, coat with the olive oil. Spread the fries evenly on a baking sheet and sprinkle with seasoned salt. Pre-heat oven to 400°F and bake for 45 minutes turning every 10 minutes. Put on medium broil for final 5 minutes for added crispness.

What Can I Do about Snacks When My Children Go to Birthday Parties?

As mentioned in an earlier chapter, if your children are eating healthily 80 percent of the time but fall off the health wagon at birthday parties or sleepovers 20 percent of the time, that is okay. It is better to let them have the occasional sweet such as cake or ice cream with their buddies than to single them out and make them feel different.

If your children have had a bad food day, put the extra effort into providing them with optimal nutrition when they return home. Fresh-squeezed fruit or vegetable juices can help a child's system recover from junk food overload. These juices can be mixed with ice in a blender to make a slushy drink that all kids love or can be frozen into healthy Popsicles. Give them plenty of fresh, clean water to help clear out their little systems.

Can Bed-wetting Be Related to Food Allergies or Sensitivities?

Yes. Food allergies and food sensitivities can be the root of the problem. If your child wets the bed, try removing dairy and wheat from his or her diet for a month. In addition, do not let your children eat a heavy meal right before bedtime because it will send them into a very deep sleep cycle, making them less likely to wake up to go to the bathroom. If they are hungry at night, give them a light snack such as a piece of fruit or a vegetable. Chiropractic care has also achieved much success with children suffering from bed-wetting.

Children who wet the bed need support, not discipline. This is not a situation in which they are acting out or being bad and need to be punished. In fact, stressful situations and unresolved emotional conflict can actually exacerbate the condition. Often children feel embarrassed by their condition and become anxious about the idea of sleepovers at a friend's house or at camp. Try to ease their stress by assuring them that they will indeed grow out of it and that every step will be taken to help stop the problem. Hugs, support, and focus on their positive attributes will help the situation.

What Should I Do When They Have a Fever?

Although most people think 98.6°F is normal body temperature, children's body temperature can range from 97–99.4°F. It is not uncommon for parents to be fever phobic and want to treat the fever immediately with Tylenol or aspirin. However, there are times when fevers are a blessing in disguise. Viruses or bacteria live at body temperature. When a fever occurs, white fighting blood cells are activated and the body temperature heats up to kill off the potentially threatening bugs. Research shows that giving a child an anti-fever drug for a low to moderate fever may actually interfere with this natural defense mechanism.

So, how high is too high and when should you treat the fever? A survey found that parents tend to treat high temperatures much more aggressively than health care professionals do. Investigators found that only 43 percent of parents (compared to 86 percent of doctors and 64 percent of nurses) knew that a fever below 100.4°F could be beneficial to a child. Most parents (compared to only 11 percent of doctors) reported that they would treat a fever below 100.4°F even if the child had no other symptoms.[2] If your children have a fever under 102°F, anti-fever medications should be used sparingly and with discretion.

One of the greatest concerns parents have about fever is the potential for a febrile seizure. While these occurrences are very frightening to watch, studies show that febrile seizures cause no long-term neurological damage and are a condition a child will grow out of. Fever-related seizures typically occur at very high temperatures (105–108°F).

When your children suffer from a fever, hydrate them well with plenty of water, natural juices, and warm broths. If they have lost their appetite for a couple of days, do not force them to eat. Loss of appetite is an adaptive response associated with fever that allows the body to deal with the problem at hand.

Should My Children Eat Fruit with Meals?

Fruit is a wonderful snack for children to munch on. However, fruit eaten with other foods can act like glue in the system. In the stomach, fruit ferments with other foods, making digestion sluggish and much more taxing on the system. Therefore, a large meal followed by a fruit-filled dessert is definitely not a good habit. Whenever possible, try to have your children eat fruit at least half an hour to an hour away from other foods.

My Children Are Very Active and Participate in Sports. Do They Need an Additional Supplement Such as Creatine to Build Muscle?

No, not if they are eating properly. Very active children will require more calories in the form of complex carbohydrates and proteins, but a supplement is not necessary. Complex carbohydrates such as whole grain breads, cereals, pasta, and bars will provide them with long-lasting fuel while high-quality proteins will ensure that muscle damage does not occur. I do not recommend that children use creatine under any circumstances. Creatine is a very common supplement used by athletes to bulk up muscle mass. Some may be under the misconception that creatine is safe and effective for athletic children, but it is not. Studies are not available on this, and adult creatine supplementation can result in serious side effects. Vegetable or whey protein powders are a safe option to add to a morning shake if desired.

Should My Teenager Wear an Antiperspirant or Deodorant?

In short, the answer is no. Antiperspirants are used to reduce perspiration, while deodorants are used to remove body odor. Although these products are used by most teens, they may be more problematic than once thought.

A teenage girl going to the gym is likely to roll on a product that contains both antiperspirant and deodorant. By doing so, she has sealed off her sweat glands, allowing toxic buildup to occur in her underarm and in close proximity to her breast.

Preliminary research is linking the use of antiperspirants and deodorants with the development of skin irritation, rashes, inflammation, underarm granulomas, and cancer. Nearly all breast cancers are located in the upper, outside quadrant where the breast and underarm lymph node tissues are located. Of course, numerous factors can contribute to breast cancer; however, the curious location of nearly all breast cancers does make one wonder if there is a link with use of antiperspirants and deodorants. Antiperspirants also contain compounds of aluminum, zinc, and zirconium while deodorants contain an antibacterial agent called triclosan, which can cause liver damage. High levels of aluminum have been indicated in the development of Alzheimer's disease.

I recommend switching your teen to a natural deodorant that will control odor while allowing the body to rid itself of toxins. Some of the best and most effective brands available at health food stores are:

- Kiss My Face
- Jason Natural Cosmetics
- Tom's of Maine
- Burt's Bees
- Nature's Gate
- Dessert Essence

TRY

1. **Picking water as the number one beverage for a child. If necessary, water down some fruit juice to sweeten. Save pop/soda as a very occasional treat.**

2. **Getting your child into the routine of taking their multi-vitamin every morning with breakfast.**

3. **Keeping a keen eye on your child's health when making nutritional changes. Subtle changes are usually noticed in children's skin, mood, energy, weight, etc. in a short amount of time.**

4. **Making your child's room an environment they enjoy and are comfortable sleeping in. Pick their favorite colors, themes and hobbies to fill their room.**

5. **Keeping the lines of conversation between you and your child constantly open. Whether you have a tot or a teenager, your ear and focus will provide a child with a safe place to go for trust and support.**

NOTES

1 www.cassmd.com
2 www.mercola.com

Palate-Pleasing Products

DAIRY ALTERNATIVES

Rice Slices: Made by Galaxy Foods; vegan, casein-free slices; other products include grated Parmesan cheese, rice sour cream, rice cream cheese, and rice butter

Tofutti Products: Dairy-free cream cheese (numerous flavors), ice cream, tofutti teddy pops, and tofutti cuties (delicious ice cream sandwiches for kids)

Veggie Slices: Made by Galaxy Foods; Italian or American flavor; they contain casein (a milk protein); however, vegan slices are available

Yves Veggie Cuisine Slices: Slices and shreds (contain soy and casein)

MEATLESS PRODUCTS

Amy's Kitchen: Texas or California burgers; are perfect for busy people who want to eat healthily. They are the top sellers of frozen natural meals such as enchiladas, vegetable potpie, lasagna, etc. The many tasty and quick options are a blessing for busy families. Available in most health food stores and some large grocery chains throughout North America

Money's Garden Burgers: Excellent, tasty garden burgers that are delicious on the barbeque

Yves Veggies Cuisine: Found in most grocery stores; a delicious assortment of meatless products available such as meatballs, hot dogs, veggie burgers, ground beef, and pepperoni. The pepperoni is wonderful on a pizza! These products are organic; however, they do contain wheat

Zoglo's: Chicken nuggets, veggie cutlets, meatless wieners, etc.; contain wheat

HEALTHY, HIGH-FIBER PASTAS, BREADS, AND MUFFINS

Eden Organic Pasta: Spinach ribbons, spinach spirals, sesame rice spirals, mixed grain spirals

Purity Food's Vita Spelt: Spelt rotini, spelt elbows, lasagna noodles, bread, pancake, and muffin mixes; spelt cookies for kids also available

Rizopia Brown Rice Pasta: Gluten-free

Tinkyada Rice Pasta: Gluten-free

HEALTHY MACARONI AND CHEESE

Amy's Kitchen: Dairy-free (soy) or with cheese

Annie's: Shells and cheddar

HEALTHY COOKIES

Country Choice: Wheat-free, milk-free, contains no hydrogenated oils, refined sweeteners, artificial flavors, colors, or preservatives. There is a large selection to choose from including double-fudge brownie, old-fashioned oatmeal, and (my personal favorite), ginger!

Frookies: Chocolate chip cookies, ginger snaps, sandwich crèmes, etc.

Healthy Times: Organic arrowroot for toddlers and organic wheat-free, dairy-free teething cookies for infants

Mi-DEL Cookies: Ginger, chocolate and lemon snaps. Made from organic flour and sweetened with cane juice.

Mrs. Denson's: Wheat-free, dairy-free, organic options including hazelnut fudge and chocolate chip macaroon

HEALTHY BARS

Cliff Bars: Chocolate brownie, chocolate almond fudge, carrot cake

Luna Bars: Orange bliss, lemon zest, toasted nuts n' cranberry

HEALTHY CHIP-LIKE SNACKS

Garden of Eatin: All-natural tortilla chips; try the sesame blues flavor!

Guiltless Gourmet: Baked, not fried, tortilla chips

Robert's American Gourmet: VEGGIE BOOTY, PIRATE'S BOOTY, SMART PUFFS, POWER PUFFS, POTATO FLYERS. These products are much healthier than hydrogenated potato chips and are perfect for a healthy snack. My nephews cannot get enough of VEGGIE BOOTY, which is loaded with immune-boosting spinach and kale.

Ruth's Hemp Tortilla Chips: Certified organic and GMO-free

HEALTHY CEREALS

Barbara's Bakery: Organic fruity punch, apple cinnamon toasted, honey nut toasted

Envirokidz Cereals: Amazon frosted flakes, Koala Crisp, Panda Puffs, etc.

Erewhon Instant Oatmeal: Apple raisin, apple cinnamon

Health Valley: Oatbran flakes

HEALTHY JUICES

Black River Juices: Flavors include Bartlett Pear, Montmorency Cherry and Concord Grape

Ceres: White grape, youngberry, papaya, strawberry, and pear

Santa Cruz: Organic lemonade

Sarah's: Apricot, banana, cranberry, blackberry

Tropicana: 100 percent orange juice

Welch's: Grape juice from concentrate

DAIRY-FREE MILKS

Edensoy

Rice Dream: Original, vanilla, chocolate

So Nice

Soy Dream

Vitasoy

Note: Similar to cow's milk, once opened, soy milk lasts for only a few days in the fridge.

ALTERNATIVE TO MAYONNAISE

Nasoya "Nayonaise": Low-fat, dairy-free mayonnaise that has 70 percent fewer calories than regular mayonnaise and is not made with "funny fats"

FAST FOOD THE "HEALTHIER" WAY

I am not advocating fast foods in children's diets. I believe they should be eliminated completely. However, the reality is that sometimes fast foods are unavoidable, so it is important to be aware of the healthier fast-food options that are now available.

Harvey's: Canadian chain; veggie burger or salads

McDonald's: Veggie burger or salads (veggie burger contains 8.2 grams of fat, whereas a Big Mac contains 32 grams of fat)

Subway: Veggie delite sub (contains only 1 gram of saturated fat)

Wendy's: Salads

NATURAL TOOTHPASTES

Dessert Essence: Herbal-Vedic (ayurvedic formulas) Jason

Nature's Gate: Cherry, mint

Tom's of Maine: Silly Strawberry flavor for kids

APPENDIX II

Healthy Bulk Bargains

The notion that health is more expensive and therefore out of the question for your family is not necessarily true. One of the greatest ways to cut costs and eat healthily at the same time is to buy in bulk! Bulk offers a wide variety of snack foods, meal options, and sweet, healthy delights for children. When I was researching for this book, I was pleased to discover that most bulk food establishments had explanations and ingredient lists attached to all the products. The following are some dollar-saving, health-promoting ideas the entire family will enjoy.

SNACK MIXES

- **Nuts:** cashews, almonds, natural pistachios, macadamia nuts, almonds, peanuts, soy nuts (barbeque, honey roasted, or regular), walnuts, pecans
- **Seeds:** pumpkin, sunflower, or sesame seeds (excellent to put into a cookie recipe!)
- **Dried fruits:** raisins, pitted dates, pitted prunes, mango slices, apple rings, papaya chunks, pineapple wedges, blueberries, cherries, or cranberries
- **Granola mixes:** berry granolas, cranberry delight granola, honey and almond granola, muesli granola, hemp granola
- **Toasted corn:** barbeque, unsalted, or salted
- **Popping corn:** air pop, sprinkle with salt, and add flaxseed oil instead of butter!

Here is an example of the ingredient list for cranberry delight granola found at the local "Bulk Barn": Oats, canola oil, spelt flour, cranberries, and currants.

Note: Although certain dried fruits contain some sugar, they are much healthier options when compared to preservative-laden chips, crackers, candy, or chocolate bars.

HEALTHY GRAINS
- Brown basmati rice
- Brown rice
- Brown rice flour
- Brown rice pasta (fettuccini, elbows, spaghetti, spirals)
- Buckwheat flour
- Dark rye flour
- Millet
- Organic brown rice cakes
- Organic quinoa
- Organic spelt flour
- Rolled oats (large or small flakes for cereal)
- Soya flour

BEANS
- Black-eyed peas
- Lima beans
- Pinto beans
- Red lentils
- Roman beans
- White and red kidney beans

OTHER HEALTHY DELIGHTS
- Spices
- Natural peanut butter
- Vegetarian chili mix
- Flaxseeds
- Textured vegetable protein
- Turbinado sugar
- Demerara sugar

APPENDIX III

A Child's Healthy Day

Breakfast	
1. FOODS	**BENEFITS**
• Multigrain, spelt, or kamut toast with natural nut butters and jam or bananas, light cream cheese, or soy cream cheese • Glass of natural orange juice or grape juice	• High in fiber • Complex carbohydrate provides long, sustaining energy Vitamin B and folate • Protein source in the cream cheese or nut butters
2. FOODS	**BENEFITS**
• Oatmeal sweetened with dates, maple syrup, raisins, or honey • Berries and ground flaxseeds drizzled over oatmeal for sweetness and crunch	• High in soluble fiber • Flaxseeds are a source of omega-3 EFA • Berries are anti-cancers (they contain bioflavonoids) • Provides long, sustaining energy
3. FOODS	**BENEFITS**
• Milkshake—soy milk, orange juice, banana, raspberries, blueberries, or strawberries; add green powder and mix in blender on high	• Protein source in the soy milk • Very filling for children wanting to lose weight • Phytonutrients in green powder • Satisfies a child's sweet tooth with natural sugars

4. FOODS	BENEFITS
• Omega-3 scrambled eggs with tomato, peppers, and mushrooms; shredded cheese or tofu cheese can be added	• Excellent protein source • High in omega-3 • Veggies contain minerals, vitamins, and phytonutrients

5. FOODS	BENEFITS
• Healthy cereals made from kamut, spelt, quinoa, or brown rice available in most health food stores and some grocery stores • Add raisins on top for sweetness	• High in fiber • Lower than refined flours on glycemic index • Long, sustaining energy source • Contains a natural source of vitamin B and folate

Lunch

1. FOODS	BENEFITS
• Avocado, hummus, tomato, and tofu cheese or goat cheese wrap • Cut-up apple slices and/or raisins • Granola bar • Bottle of water	• Goat or soy cheese are good sources of protein • Wrap will provide some fiber • Apple contains fiber, bioflavonoids, and natural enzymes for digestion • Nuts and seeds in granola bar contain omega-3 EFA

2. FOODS	BENEFITS
• Natural peanut butter and jam sandwich on multigrain, kamut, or spelt bread • Carrots and celery • Healthier cookie selection (such as "Frookies," available at most health food stores) • Bottle of water	• Frookie satisfies child's desire for a "treat" • Carrots contain beta-carotene • Bread selection contains vitamin B and folate • Nut butters are a good source of protein

3. FOODS	BENEFITS
• Tuna on brown rice bread with tomato sauce and melted soy, rice, or goat cheese • Carrots and broccoli dipped in hummus or salsa • 1 homemade chocolate chip cookie • Bottle of water	• Tuna contains omega-3 and is an excellent source of protein • Brown rice bread provides an excellent source of fuel for the body and is rich in vitamin B and folate • Carrots and broccoli are loaded with calcium and vitamin C
4. FOODS	**BENEFITS**
• Healthy macaroni and cheese made from soy or cow's cheese • Corn and bean salad • Naturally sweetened apple sauce	• Macaroni noodles are a good source of fuel that will not cause blood sugar to fluctuate • Beans are a good source of fiber • Apple sauce contains some vitamin C, fiber, and natural enzymes
5. FOODS	**BENEFITS**
• Healthy grilled cheese sandwich on multigrain bread with organic dairy, soy or rice cheese • Sliced oranges and bananas	• Bread provides fuel, B vitamins, folate and fiber • Bananas and oranges provide vitamin C, potassium, and help kids to increase their live food intake

Dinner

1. FOODS	BENEFITS
• Healthy Taco Night—shredded cheese (soy or dairy), tomato, lettuce, with sliced chicken or veggie ground round (imitation meat product by Yves Veggie Cuisine), and salsa • Spinach salad with dressing made from flaxseed oil • Bottle of water	• Tortillas shells are an excellent source of calcium • Veggie ground round or chicken are good protein selections • Spinach provides absorbable calcium, vitamin C, folic acid, and numerous minerals • Flaxseed for its omega-3 value

2. FOODS	BENEFITS
• Kamut, spelt, or brown rice pasta with tomato sauce (Parmesan or dairy-free Parmesan on top is optional) • Lightly steamed and seasoned broccoli with optional melted soy or organic cow or goat cheese on top • Bottle of water	• The bread is high in complex carbohydrates • Tomatoes contain lycopene, a powerful anti-cancer element • Broccoli is a "green powerhouse" packed with calcium and vitamin C • Soy contains cancer-fighting substances called phytoestrogens

3. FOODS	BENEFITS
• Spelt pizza crust with tomato sauce, veggie pepperoni (from Yves Veggie Cuisine), pineapple, and onions • Bottle of water	• Pineapple contains natural digestive enzymes called bromelain • Spelt pizza crust is a healthy, non-processed complex carbohydrate • Yves veggie pepperoni contains an excellent source of protein

4. FOODS	BENEFITS
• Veggie or salmon burger on a brown rice bun • Cut-up tomatoes and pickles • Yam French fries, sliced and baked in oven • Condiment of choice • Bottle of water	• Salmon or veggie burger are good sources of protein • Salmon is an excellent source of omega-3 • Yams contain carotenes and vitamin C

5. FOODS	BENEFITS
• Vegetarian or chicken chili—include navy beans, lentils, broccoli, peppers, tomatoes, tomato sauce, and season to taste • Add sprinkled cheese on top if so desired • Multigrain bread to dip into chili • Bottle of water	• Beans are an excellent source of fiber and protein and are very filling • Chicken fulfils protein requirement • Multigrain bread will ensure blood sugar levels are stabilized

Healthy sweet snack ideas

- Healthy trail mix of raw seeds, nuts, and raisins for sweetness
- Baked nachos or chips dipped into salsa
- Veggie Bootie (a chip-like snack filled with kale and rice—kids love it!)
- Naturally sweetened yogurt or pudding (such as Imagine Pudding)
- Naturally sweetened applesauce
- A healthy granola bar
- Soy ice cream or ice cream sandwiches (such as Tofutti Cuties)
- Homemade cinnamon oatmeal cookies sweetened with maple syrup or applesauce
- Dried apricots or apples
- Naturally sweetened dark chocolate squares
- Veggies and dip such as guacamole, hummus, or ranch dip
- Barbeque or salt and vinegar soybeans

Dr. Joey's Top Supplement Picks for Kids

1. greens+ kids

2. o3mega

3. Acidophilus – ensure brand you are purchasing has a minimum of 1 billion organisms

FOR MORE INFORMATION ON PRODUCTS LISTED IN THIS BOOK:

- greens+ kids: www.greenspluscanada.com
- Whole Foods Market: large grocery and health food chain throughout North America, www.wholefoods.com

SUPPLEMENTS FOR HEALING

These supplements will reduce the inflammation and correct an underlying problem. Even if your children are on an anti-inflammatory drug such as corticosteroids, the supplements will help to heal the bowel and make weaning children off the medication easier. *Speak to your doctor before making any medication changes in your children.* Corticosteroids cannot just be stopped. Dosages must be reduced gradually under the supervision of your primary health practitioner.

- **Acidophilus and bifidus:** These "friendly bacteria" are necessary to restore proper digestion and normalize bowel function. This supplement should be taken on an empty stomach, twice daily as directed on the bottle. Purchase a product that contains at least 1 billion organisms.

- **Omega-3 essential fatty acid:** These healing oils repair the intestinal tract and reduce inflammation. Similar to a conditioner coating a hair follicle, omega-3 oil and its derivative, DHA, will coat and repair the intestinal wall. Essential fatty acids such as omega-3 also help rebuild cells in the body and are necessary for providing energy. Put 1–2 tablespoons a day in your children's juice, applesauce, pudding, or shake. If they are old enough, they can take capsules. Due to a child's compromised digestive state, I recommend using fish, not flax oil for this condition.

- **Digestive enzymes (chewable):** Enzymes are molecules (usually proteins) that assist in the breakdown of carbohydrates, fats, proteins, and fiber, thereby enhancing digestion. Children suffering from IBD need to have their food broken down sufficiently to allow their digestive system the chance to heal. I recommend taking two digestive enzymes directly before each meal. If your children suffer from arthritis related to Crohn's or colitis, also give them digestive enzymes between meals (up to twelve per day). Enzymes taken with food help digest the food; enzymes taken between meals "munch up" harmful microorganisms, reducing inflammation and arthritis symptoms.

- **Green powder:** Because children with IBD must avoid certain foods and are unable to digest properly, they are at risk of suffering from malnourishment. While healing is taking place, it is wise to supplement with a green powder filled with essential nutrients Since most children with IBD are unable to eat raw fruits and vegetables for a while, this supplement will give them the extra boost they need.

Studies have shown that 30–60 percent of IBD patients may have low bone density.

- **Calcium/magnesium supplement (liquid if possible):** Magnesium is helpful in relaxing the intestinal wall and decreasing the cramping and pain. Children require a daily intake of 6 milligrams of magnesium per pound of body weight. For example, a five-year-old requires approximately 240 milligrams daily, while a twelve-year-old requires 600 milligrams daily.[1] Liquid supplementation is best in order to increase absorption. If your children are having difficulty sleeping, a calcium/magnesium supplement given at bedtime can be helpful.

"Before meeting Dr. Joey, my life was filled with stomach pain, cramps, bleeding, and severe bowel movements. I would have to plan my activities according to how my stomach was feeling and how my Crohn's disease was at the time. Five years and four major surgeries later, I went to see Dr. Joey. It is thanks to her that I have my life back. She taught me how to help myself through the foods I eat. She took the time to explain to me why the changes were necessary and why it was important to stick with the dietary changes. The only regret I have is not seeing her sooner because I know that with her help, I could have probably avoided surgery. (Saying) thank you will never be enough to express the gratitude that I feel toward Dr. Joey. I recommend her to everyone that I know that suffers from bowel disorders. Thanks a million.

—CAROLINE SAMSON, Ontario

NOTES

1 L. Galland, *Superimmunity for Kids* (New York: Dell Publishing, 1989).

Index